Hidden Secrets
For
Better Vision

An in-depth glance into the latest
breakthrough research and wisdom for the
successful treatment of eye disorders
and vision problems.

Fischer Publishing Corporation
Canfield, Ohio 44406

Disclaimer

Medical information presented in this book *Hidden Secrets For Better Vision* is furnished by accredited opthalmic authority, Leslie H. Salov, M.D., O.D., Ph.D. While Leslie H. Salov, M.D., O.D., Ph. D. and William L. Fischer are collaborating here as co-authors, Dr. Salov is the eye-care expert, and William L. Fischer is the medical journalist reporting on such information.

If you, as a potential user of information found on these pages, require opinions, diagnoses, treatments, or any other aid relating to vision, it is recommended by the publisher that you consult either Dr. Leslie H. Salov, or your own eye specialist.

Nothing noted in the text should be considered an attempt by William L. Fischer or the publisher to practice medicine, prescribe remedies, make diagnoses or act as persuasion for enforcing some mode of self treatment.

Instead, knowledge received is strictly for purposes of education, and William L. Fischer takes no responsibility for its vision care content.

TABLE OF CONTENTS

FOREWORD

Today more people than ever before realize that the adage "you are what your eat" is true. Nutrient intake plays a large role in determining the state of our health. Physicians have long known that a diet lacking in iron, eventually, will produce anemia in a person. And it is common knowledge, for example, that diet has been identified as a major factor in such deadly conditions as heart disease and some types of cancer. But health professionals have only recently acknowledged that diet, and especially proper nutrient intake, influence the health of the eyes.

Vitamin and mineral deficiencies can cause potentially serious problems with the eyes, ranging from night blindness to cataracts. Cataracts, for example, were once thought to be an unavoidable part of the aging process. Now, many researchers have discovered that in certain cases, the formation of the cloudy lens may be due to a deficiency of specific nutrients.

The most advanced research is showing, moreover, that supplementation with Vitamin C has been helpful in the prevention of cataracts for some people. Nutritionists echo these sentiments, saying that a life-long, well-balanced diet, may save your eyesight.

In *Hidden Secrets For Better Vision,* Dr. Leslie Salov and William L. Fischer explore the realm of nutrition and eyesight, from vitamins that may help improve your night vision to minerals that may actually reduce your risk of becoming a victim of macular degeneration. They also present symptoms of various eye conditions from the rare to the commonplace. Knowing these warning signs of diseases may save your sight or that of a loved one.

Alternatives to Myopia

Think you're struck with those eyeglasses you've been wearing since childhood? Think again. Consider the near miraculous, new, painless procedure, radial keratotomy, in which one can rediscover the joys of perfect 20/20 vision again. Or for a more natural way back to good eyesight, examine MacKay's presentation of the Bates method for eye exercises. The exercises provided have restored eyesight to many who felt they had been condemned to a lifetime depending on eyeglasses.

While a person, naturally, is constantly using his eyes, continued reading or television watching causes one not to fully utilize all of the eye muscles. It is important, adherents of the Bates method assert, that one change focus as much as possible. By switching the point of focus from nearby to distant objects regularly, all of the eye muscles are exercised. Just as your leg muscles need a variety of movements to stay strong and healthy, your eyes also need similar consideration.

Included in this book are several exercises to familiarize yourself with the Bates method and Dr. Salov's therapies as well as the address of the organization's national center. The people there will provide you with more information as well as help you locate an experienced eye therapist in your area, if you desire more instruction.

Dr. Salov and William Fischer have written a well-researched, comprehensive book on the health of the eyes. Every person, no matter his age or range of vision should read this book to discover the hidden secrets to having healthy eyes.

John MacKay

INTRODUCTION

Look around you. Count the number of people today who wear eyeglasses. An astonishingly high number of people need the ocular crutches to perform even the simplest of daily duties. Many confess that their eyeglasses are the first thing they reach for every morning upon arising. How else could they see their alarm clock?

It's a sad state of affairs. People who consider themselves otherwise healthy tolerate a deplorable state of health for their eyes. What's even sadder is the complacency, not of the public at large, but of the medical profession. Too many doctors in the past have accepted the notion there is nothing one can do to to improve his eyesight. Too many ophthalmologists view the cataract formation as just one of the penalties of growing old. Blind acceptance of these notions has created a danger-ous pattern of thought and approach to the prob-lem.

Previously, conventional wisdom dictated that a person who suffers from myopia was condemned to a lifetime of wearing glasses. And, after he reached the age of 40, the odds were highly stacked that he would need bifocals. Presbyopia—the less-ened ability of the eye to focus at close range—is one of the consequences of aging, eye doctors said, shrugging their shoulders.

Fortunately, conventional wisdom is changing. Researchers are successfully challenging the old ideas, providing new hypotheses as well as the data to substantiate them. It's a rapidly changing world of facts when it comes to the human eye. What causes myopia? What causes cataracts and glaucoma? Can they be prevented?

This book is dedicated to helping you discover the answers to questions like these. Think of *Hidden Secrets For Better Vision* as a scorecard on the volumes of research the medical community has been producing in recent years. It brings together not only the latest nutritional research pertaining to eyesight and the very latest in surgical techniques, but it also offers the wisdom of generations past, in the form of herbal remedies for many of the ailments of the eye.

Remedies to Myopia

First, let's talk briefly about myopia, commonly called nearsightedness. A portion of this book is devoted to explaining the success of the painless procedure of radial keratotomy, an amazing operation which can eliminate nearsightedness. Developed abroad, the surgery has gained the acceptance of the medical community as an alternative to wearing either eyeglasses or contact lenses.

Many former nearsighted people have found new lives because of this marvelous procedure. We share their stories with you, because they are average people just like you and we are. The only difference is their lives have been touched by an extraordinary medical advance.

We have also devoted a chapter to a natural method of restoring eyesight — the Bates Exercise System. A system pioneered and named after New York ophthalmologist, William Bates, the eye exercises provide the muscles of the eye with proper and systematic movements. Bates and his followers say that the average person does not use his eye muscles to the fullest extent possible. Activities such as reading or television viewing, which almost demands that a person gaze for extended periods of time without shifting his focus may lead to the loss of muscle tone.

The solution, according to this popular school of thought, is the regular changing of one's focus from objects nearby to those at a distance. In this way one uses the full range of the eye's capabilities.

Don't let the simplicity of the eye exercises deceive you. People have reported permanent improvement in their eyesight by following the

Bates drills. We've included some of the more important and effective ones. In fact, while researching the topic, we began a conscious effort to follow some of the advice Bates' adherents offer. One of the ways to improve eyesight was not to allow your eyes to focus on any single object for more than a minute. If one is reading, try quickly looking up every so often and focus on a distant object.

Indeed, after four hours of intensive library work, the eyes feel great, not tired as had been anticipated. And what was remarkable, was that distant signs in the library could be read more clearly than before.

Nutrition and The Eye

The health of the eye is not an isolated condition, separate from the status of the rest of your body. No, the state of the eye reflects the general health of the whole system. Therefore, the eye reacts to nutrient deficiencies in the same manner as other organs of the body.

Indeed, more researchers are investigating the fact that a lack of certain vitamins may help promote the formation of cataracts, the single leading cause of blindness in the United States. And there's evidence that a diet high in refined sugar may also help speed the formation of the cloudy lenses.

It seems so logical that nutrition is a key to eye health—Vitamin A, for instance, has long been associated with battling night blindness—that one wonders why research in this field is just in its infancy. Nonetheless, the results are nothing less than exciting. A nutritional focus on the health of the eye offers people a natural way of correcting vision and eliminating conditions previously handled exclusively through synthetic drugs or surgery. A step toward the natural is welcome, indeed.

Artificial Light

Among the many discoveries we made during the research for this book was the realization that today, the average person spends the majority of his time under artificial lights. This situation poses problems, experts are now discovering, in a wide range of areas — including problems for the eyes.

Incandescent light—the light emitted from a regular household bulb—has long been with us. Researchers consider it causes little problems. Rather, the continued exposure to fluorescent light, which is the type the vast majority of us work under every day in the office or plant, seems to be the worst type of light for us.

Sunlight emits a wide range of rays, some visible and some invisible, which suits the needs of the human body quite nicely. Fluorescent light does not produce the entire spectrum of rays and of those emitted, some are not in the proper proportion for the continued good of our health. This, it seems, say the experts in the field, is causing problems with, not only our health, but also our behavior. Be sure to read this chapter and discover the differences in children's attitudes, grades and behavior when observed working under fluorescent light and the more natural full spectrum fluorescent lighting. There are many examples of full spectrum light advantages. We have chosen two schools from North America to illustrate the point. Full spectrum light, in addition to saving one's eyesight, may help boost achievement and may even prevent cavities.

Dr. Leslie Salov
William L. Fischer

Chapter 1

Your Windows To The World

A 45-year-old man, president of his own billion-dollar independent oil exploration and refining company, Kenneth Getwell, Jr. of Houston, Texas, had exceedingly poor vision. In each eye the man had minus five diopters of nearsightedness, which gave him uncorrected vision of 20/400. It was necessary for him to wear eyeglasses during his waking moments, since without them Getwell couldn't even count fingers held in front of his face.

In February 1984, the oil multimillionaire, a devoted family man, took his wife and three children to Acapulco for a weekend jaunt. Among them was his favorite offspring, little Georgie, age six, who loved to swim and jump in the waves. Getwell enjoyed watching the youngster play in the water.

The only time the former wildcatter removed his spectacles during daylight activities was when he went swimming himself. Of course, without corrective lenses the man couldn't see any kind of detail, just color differentiations among various shapes.

On this bright December afternoon gamboling on the beach and in the azure blue waters of the vacation resort, Getwell and Georgie were cherishing some time alone together. Nobody else was on their particular stretch of beach. Georgie ran into the waves and swam out to the open water. The father, seeing this, let the little boy go for a short distance. Then he became somewhat alarmed because he knew his young son was in water well over his head. The man called for the child to turn back, but Georgie apparently did not hear.

Methodically, Getwell removed his shirt, sneakers, and eyeglasses, tucked the spectacles safely into a tennis shoe, and stepped into the water. He couldn't see anything much but did swim in the general direction where he thought Georgie to be. He swam and swam but seemed never to reach the boy. Getwell couldn't see him or hear him; the tyke had just disappeared, and the father felt panic.

His eyes focused better underwater than in the air, since water magnifies underwater by 25 percent. Getwell spotted a dark spot about eight feet below him and dived toward it. It happened that the dark object was his son, whom he grabbed up and brought in to shore. The child was unhurt but thoroughly frightened. It had been his first experience with hazardous currents and undertow.

Getwell and his family were quite disturbed by this incident, which could be indirectly attributed to the father's nearsightedness. As soon as he returned home, the man went to visit Warren D. Cross, M.D., an outstanding ophthalmologist who conducts eye surgery practices in two separate locations in Houston, Bellaire Eye Associates and Town and Country Eye Associates. Getwell told Dr. Cross that his myopic eyes were rather ineffective windows to the world, and he never wanted any accident similar to Acapulco's to happen again. His preference was for permanent surgical correction of the five-diopter nearsightedness.

Using a high-tech vision technique, Dr. Cross performed the patient's required refractive correction in one of his Houston-area offices. It was a highly successful operation. Following postoperative healing, Kenneth Getwell, Jr. was able to see with perfect 20/20 vision. Wearing eyeglasses became totally unnecessary for the oil man, and he proceeded to throw them away. More complete pictures of the world now entered through his visual windows.

What Makes Normal 20/20 Vision?

The description of Mr. Getwell achieving 20/20

3

vision means that his eyes now see at 20 feet what any normal eyes can see at 20 feet. The ratio of 20 to 20 refers to the difference between the eye being measured and a theoretical normal-seeing eye. For example, if you are told by your eye doctor that you have 20/40 vision in the left eye, that eye has to be as close as 20 feet to see what a normal eye can see at 40 feet. It has about one half normal vision. Remember, Getwell was corrected from myopic vision of 20/400.

On the other hand, if your right eye is 20/15, that means it can see at 20 feet what normal eye sees when placed within 15 feet of an object. It has vision approximately 25 percent better than normal. When the anatomy of the eye is functioning physiologically correctly, you are able to see with 20/20 vision.

In this chapter, we will briefly describe the many components which comprise the eye's functional anatomy - parts of the eye providing normal 20/20 vision. Please refer to the accompanying diagrams of the eye's components for clarification of the anatomy.

The central area in the eye furnishing the best sight is the *macula*, which is some 1/20th of an inch in diameter. The macula contains most of the 6.25 million cones that join together with 125 million rods which make up the approximately

130,000,000 light-sensitive cells in the retina. Retinal *cones* are specialized visual cells responsible for sharpness of vision and color vision. Retinal *rods* respond to light, dark, movements, shapes, but not to colors.

The very tightest concentration of cones (147,000 per square millimeter (mm)) is the *fovea,* a tiny depression in the center of the macula. When you look at something you turn your eyes so that the light rays are focused precisely on the fovea. There is very little overlying tissue to block the light rays.

The *retina* is the lining at the back of the eye where the image is formed. It is composed of those specialized light-sensitive cells that we've mentioned, rods and cones, plus various typical brain-type cells, and a network of a formidable complex system of interconnected nerve cells. Its rods share a common line to the brain. The more numerous the rods are distributed throughout the retina, the number getting fewer at the extreme edges.

Along with the retina, crammed into the *eyeball,* which is a sphere about an inch long, are other specialized parts. The *cornea* is a transparent tissue covering the front of the eye much as a watch crystal covers a watch, except that it is living tissue. The cornea is clear as crystal and situated in front of the iris and pupil.

The *iris* is a thin circular curtain which is the

colored part of the eye. A person's eye color depends on the amount of pigment in the iris; deep brown eyes have the most pigment and light blue have the least.

The *pupil* is a hole in the center of the iris. It is black because the inside of the eye is dark. The pupil's size varies with the amount of light entering, for it can get smaller with increased light and larger with lessened light.

The tough, but delicate and sensitive outer coat of the eye, actually is composed of two parts. As mentioned, the cornea is one, and the sclera is the other. The *sclera* is opaque (impervious to light) and protects the rest of the eye: it's referred to as the "white of the eye."

The cornea is so clear from its precise alignment of fibers that unless you look closely you aren't aware of its presence. If any interference occurs in the fibers' orderly alignment, the cornea gets cloudy and blurs the vision. This may happen from injury, scarring, or disease. The blink reflex and the lid tend to protect the cornea by their sensitivity to the slightest touch or threat of a touch. The blink instantly wipes off anything which lands on the cornea such as dust. On the other hand, if something does trouble the cornea, one feels acute pain which is a warning to get help. Loss of this sensitivity or loss of the blink reflex or of the lid action makes the cornea vulnerable to injury, covering the cornea with a contact lens might lose the eye's sensitivity, blink, or lid action.

Sometimes corneas are transplanted to replace the clouding of a diseased one. Corneas for transplantation may have been donated prior to death by considerate people.*

Lying between the sclera and the retina is a maze of blood vessels that bring nourishment to the rods and cones of the retina. This maze is called the *choroid* (pronounced KOH-royd).

A transparent, semi-soft material about half the size of a ten-cent piece - the *lens*-is able to change shape to focus on objects at different distances from the eye. The lens is held in place by threadlike *zonular* fibers, which are connected from the lens edges to tiny but powerful *ciliary* muscles. At the command of a nerve coming from the brain, the ciliary muscles tighten or loosen the zonular fibers. The lens, which is flexible, changes its shape just enough to focus the eye for far or near distances.

As the lens ages, it loses some of its flexibility. Focusing on close objects becomes difficult since the lens won't bulge as well, and presbyopia sets in. That's why some people after the age of forty require reading glasses.

*You could choose to donate your corneas upon death by simply registering with a local Eye Bank or with the Eye Bank for Sight Restoration, 210 East 46th Street, New York, New York 10021.

During the waking hours, tear fluid is produced constantly. It is a natural washer of the lens with lysozyme, a powerful germ killer. When not needed, the tear gland shuts off the tear fluid, such as during sleep.

The front and rear chambers of the eye are filled with a clear fluid called the aqueous humor. The *aqueous humor* is a crystal-clear liquid. It is able to escape from the eye if pressure is applied, and yet under normal conditions it remains constant in amount and so keeps the intraocular pressure essentially uniform. The lens, and to some extent the cornea, are devoid of blood vessels, so that their nourishment must be supplied largely by the bathing fluid, and waste products must be carried away in a similar fashion. The aqueous humor must therefore contain the building blocks necessary for tissue replacement. Such building blocks might be glucose, coenzymes, minerals, and amino acids. The aqueous humor has to transport oxygen and carry away the waste products of metabolism, including carbon dioxide, from the interior of the eye to the blood.

This same fluid permeates the gel-like substance filling the rear cavity of the eye, which is named the *vitreous humor*. The vitreous humor is regarded by eye anatomists as an intricate fibrous network supporting an optically empty fluid surrounded by a definite membrane, which separates

8

the vitreous from the lens and from the retina. In the jellylike material the same wavy gossamer-like threads or curtains can be identified at repeated slit-lamp examinations.

A ray of light passing directly from the object you see to the retina is on a line called the *visual axis.* It runs through a perfectly clear series of structures so that no light is lost and no distortion or obstruction of the image takes place. These clear structures are called the *optical media,* and they are as we describe them, from the front to the back of the eye, the cornea, the aqueous fluid, the lens, and the vitreous fluid.

How We See

We look at a dog - a German shepherd - and we "see" it; its muzzle, lolling tongue, black nose, two pointed ears, four long legs, single furry tail, lithe body, barrel chest, smooth flanks, and shiny brown with black coat. If it's our pet, the dog has recognizable reality. Yet all that our eyes have received from this animal figure is reflected light. With no light being present to reflect off the animal, we would have seen no German shepherd.

The reflected light from the dog is focused on the retina to produce patterns of electrochemical discharges which are sent to the brain in the form of nerve signals. "Seeing" the animal has us receiving a complex arrangement of coded signals that the brain interprets, recognizes, and translates into information. The information gets projected into the conscious in the form of a picture. Thus, what is seen is the characteristic and specific perceptual response we have to a particular pattern of visual impulses.

In other words, the eye is a collector of light from particular objects and translates the light into patterns of nerve signals, which the brain then interprets and pictures for the consciousness. Really, it is the brain and not the eye that does the seeing. The brain processes data with inputs, outputs, storage area, and stored duplicates, just like a computer. During an average second of its activity, the brain performs approximately five trillion operations, each one of which is associated with the discharge of an electrochemical impulse involving the five senses and the body's metabolism.

When light waves come into the eye they must be bent or refracted. *Refraction* is the change in direction of light rays when they pass obliquely from one transparent medium to another, of a different density. Refraction occurs as light enters the eye, when it passes from air to the media of the eye. It goes from the cornea to the aqueous humor to the lens to the vitreous humor to come to a focus on the retina. Errors of refraction, in which light rays do not come to a focus on the retina due to defects in the refracting media or shape of the eyeball, include such eye disabilities as nearsightedness, farsightedness, and astigmatism.

We will discuss the separate refraction disabilities including their individualized causes when we present details about their respective corrective procedures.

How clearly you see is called *acuity*. But good vision is much more of optical brain skills. Ask yourself the following questions and check your visual skills to find the answers only you can supply:

1. How well can I use both eyes together?

2. How quickly can I judge left from right?

3. How well do I see objects in space?

4. Am I able to shift focus from near to far quickly and easily - within fractions of a second?

5. How retentive is my visual memory?

6. How easily can I change my point of view?

7. Are my visual skills equal to my age and my needs?

8. How well do I check for the absence of eye disease

11

and acuity on an eye chart?

9. Am I able to get out the good ideas formed in my mind and act on them, or do they get blocked by an inefficient visual system I've suspected has been my creative problem.

10. Might visual problems be making me cranky or rigid in my outlook or cause me to seem less intelligent than I am?

Approximately 55 percent of the American population today wears eyeglasses or contact lenses for something more than being fashionable. The use of such external eye aids is equivalent to propping up vision with crutches, braces, wheel chairs, and corsets. Wearing eyeglasses or contacts is in the same league with using dentures, arch supports, hearing aids, molded shoes, and hernia belts. Yet, only about 2-1/2 percent of children are born with true visual deformities. Eye problems seem to be programmed into the human species by the high technology all of us have exposure to.

How we see is largely affected by imperfections built into the eye anatomy. Although in the previous subsection we described components of the normal eye, there is no "perfect" eye. In fact, if you were sold a camera with all the built-in imperfections of the eye, you would likely return to the photography store demanding a refund. Your first developed photographs - using the eye as your camera - would probably be full of distortions.

Focusing Light Rays to See

Employing the cornea, aqueous fluid, iris with its pupil, the lens with its ciliary body, and the vitreous humor - all the structures in front of the retina - the eye automatically focuses light rays. Focusing merely means changing the direction of light to alter the straightness of its rays (or bend it). Another word for focusing is "refraction," the act of bending a beam of light when it travels from a less dense medium to a more dense medium and vice versa. A light beam is a column of light rays moving parallel to each other in a straight line. The rays come from the sun at a speed of 186,000 miles per second. When the beam comes near to the earth, our denser atmosphere slows the speed, and upon entering your eye, the light is held back even more because of the eye's greater density.

Striking denser surfaces still, such as glass, there is even more bending of the rays, especially if they hit the surface obliquely. Nearer rays reach the surface sooner than more distant rays, causing the beam to sharply change its direction. This bending is the "refraction" we have spoken about.

13

A glass prism bends the light twice, first as it enters and again when it emerges from the glass.

Two prisms, placed base to base, will each bend rays toward its base so that they converge and focus the light at a certain distance from them. A convex lens is similar to a pair of prisms, but the lens has curved surfaces instead of straight ones. It acts like two prisms, base to base. It brings the light rays into focus. The more sharply curved the lens is, the more the light rays will converge and the closer to the lens will be the point where all the rays meet (come into focus).

Having three focusing surfaces, the eye converges light rays from (a) the front curved surface of the cornea, (b) the front curved surface of the lens, and (c) the back curved surface of the lens. The focus is supposed to fall on the retina at the back of the eyeball. The eye's lens is convex and converges light rays together to focus it just right on the retina in a normal eye. When convergence is just right, refraction is considered perfect. Sometimes it does not focus well, and then there is "error of refraction" we have mentioned previously.

Eye surgery is exceedingly well established as a medical practice. Nearly 5,000 years ago, the Code *of Hammurabi* about 1700 B.C. laid down stiff penalties for the physician whose treatment caused the loss of a patient's eye. It declared that when a freeman's eye was lost, the surgeon's fingers should be cut off, when the slave's eye was lost, the surgeon had to pay half the price of that slave. But surgeons who saved a man's eye received the same fee that was paid to a doctor who saved a life.

Miscellaneous Facts About Our Windows to the World

A recently conducted Gallup survey asked people which of the six human disabilities - blindness, muteness, limb loss, deafness, loss of smell, loss of taste - was the "worst thing that can happen to you." Of the respondents 76 percent replied blindness was the worst, which was far ahead of the next worst (9 percent selected muteness). In another survey asking about degenerative diseases, people were questioned about which affliction they dreaded most: cancer, blindness, deafness, heart disease, tuberculosis, polio, arthritis, etc. Only cancer out ranked blindness as the most terrible disorder to experience.

Almost two million Americans can't see well enough with either eye, even with corrective lenses, to read this page. Another four million have only partial vision. Ten million suffer from significant uncorrectable visual impairments which we shall discuss in Chapter Three. Approximately 15 percent to all patients treated at the nation's medical

15

centers and hospitals are eye patients. In the vicinity of 750,000 major eye operations are performed in the United States every year. Over 100 million Americans wear eyeglasses or contact lenses today. At least 30 percent of these people could throw away their external eye aids if they undertook the refractive eye corrections that the author will be describing in the following chapters.

The loss or reduction of sight impoverishes human relationships by eliminating non-verbal communication, including all forms of body language. This reduced means of communicating along with not visualizing scenes, colors, and having visual memories for retention are the subconscious fears of those who may eventually be less able to see. Every person recognizes, at least psychologically, that the eyes are your very special and irreplaceable windows to the world.

But sight and vision are not the same thing. Sight is what takes place in your eyes when you see light; *vision* is what occurs when the messages triggered by that light race through the optic nerve into the depths of your brain at an incredible 300 miles per hour. You really "see" in the visual center of the brain's cortex. The visual process consists of light, sight, vision, the eye, the optic nerve, and the visual cortex.

Just like the lens in a camera, our eye lens

produces an upside-down image on the retina; yet the brain manages to see everything right side up. The retina varies in color from a bright yellow to a very dark red, depending on the amount of pigment or color in both the choroid and the retina. Although it is onionskin thin, the retina still has thin layers of cells containing rods and cones, and the optic nerve. There are tens of millions of nerve connections in the retina handling some 1-1/2 million simultaneous impulses or messages.

Of the various operative procedures we are providing information on here, all of them are aimed at correcting the cornea. The cornea is composed of five layers of tissue, one of which consists of 300 plates with collagen fibers running through it. Yet the cornea is uniformly thick, absolutely transparent, and with cells that shed continuously to be replaced by new cells from the innermost layer. Its nutrition comes out from its own blood vessels, since none is present in healthy corneal tissue. Instead, nutrition derives from blood vessels surrounding the junction of the sclera, the aqueous humor, the tears, and the oxygen out of the air. If damage to the cornea is minor, such as a scratch, the growth and replacement that goes on will rapidly restore it to normal.

Running around the cornea and sclera is a channel the *canal of Schlemm*, which drains off the

17

excess aqueous humor and empties it through a whole system of tiny channels into the anterior ciliary vein. When this drainage systems gets blocked, glaucoma occurs.

Chapter 2

Controversies In Eye Care

Next to the brain, the eye is the most complex organ in the human body. Like any delicate and enormously intricate human body mechanism, unfortunately, the eye does not always function properly. Almost half a million people in the United States are legally blind and many others suffer from a wide range of visual disorders. They are especially subjected to refractive problems including myopia, hyperopia, presbyopia, and/or astigmatism.

Over the past decade, dramatic breakthroughs have been made in medical scientists' understanding of the eye. Vision experts are attaining more knowledge concerning the cause of eye difficulties, new scientific instruments to help detect eye trouble have been developed, and meaningful breakthroughs entailing surgical techniques to cure visual disorders have taken place. Yet, with all the breakthroughs in a diversity of eye care fields,

19

controversy among people rendering professional health care services has arisen. Competition is keen. Sometimes the many contentions, particularly between optometrists and ophthalmologists or between optometrists and opticians or among opposing groups within the separate professions themselves are bitter and combative.

Disagreements among these eye care professionals, in particular those who treat refractive problems, are based upon the von Helmholtz theory. About 126 years ago Herman Ludwig Ferdinand von Helmholtz, M.S., the inventor of the ophthalmoscope, came up with the concept of accommodation on which orthodox ophthalmology and optometry are founded. Dr. von Helmholtz claimed that accommodation is effected by the change in shape of the lens. In turn, this change is governed by the action of the ciliary muscles, although he did not offer any reasonable explanation as to how the ciliary muscles operated. He also admitted that his theory was merely a probability because the image obtained on the lens was so variable and uncertain that to use his own words, it is "most usually so blurred that the form of the flame could not be definitely distinguished."

Dr. von Helmholtz declared that nearsightedness and farsightedness, as well as most other errors of refraction, were fixed states. He stated unequivocally that these conditions could not be corrected. He believed that somewhere along the line either through birth or another reason these faults existed and there just was no cure for the situation. The only means of help, von Helmholtz said, was to wear artificial lenses so ground as to counteract the refractive error of the crystalline lens. As indicated by the operative corrections we are discussing in this book, the doctor was obviously wrong.

From the time of Dr. von Helmholtz's statement to now, the entire medical profession and its various branches dealing with vision, such as opthalmologists, opticians, and optometrists have accepted and followed the long standing principle. Millions of people around the world today wear lens corrections because of the von Helmholtz theory. Furthermore, the intraprofessional and interprofessional controversies arising from the theory's interpretation for treatment have tended to alienate colleagues from each other.

Choosing the Eye Care Professional

When a person seeking eye-care treatment walks into a professional office he is only concerned about getting the best possible servicing of his problem. But the patient would have to be an astute pupil of politics to understand the forces now at work shaping the future of the eye-care industry.

The truth is that with all of the diagnostic advances, the improved quality of eye care, and the many breakthroughs we are describing here, the competition grows among health care professionals administering to patients with vision problems. Consumers may become confused by the lobbying and heated discussions among the three groups of specialists: ophthalmologists, optometrists, and opticians. There is a basic economic conflict on various levels among the three groups, and there tends to be financial pressure from one group to downgrade the others. These various pressures, along with medical and professional concerns, account for much of the competition.

One problem that confuses consumers is choosing an eye care professional to visit regularly. An ophthalmologist (pronounced off/THAL/mol/ogist) is an eye physician and surgeon with a M.D. degree, who also is known as an oculist. This medical doctor specializes in the total care of the eyes. He or she is the only practitioner medically trained and qualified to diagnose and treat all eye and visual system problems as well as general diseases of the body. By looking within your eye, an ophthalmologist can see the signs of many systemic diseases which require immediate treatment, including diabetes, high blood pressure, and cancer.

With an instrument called a tonometer, an ophthalmologist can determine a patient's eye pressure, the force with which the fluids of the eye press against the optic nerve. High eye pressure, like high blood pressure, is a serious matter. It may indicate the presence of glaucoma.

"You have to think of the eyes in terms of the entire body," said the former president of the American Association of Ophthalmology, Alfonse Cinotti, M.D. "Prescribing corrective glasses and contact lenses is only a part of total eye care. A medical eye examination by an ophthalmologist can reveal subtle changes in your eyes which often signal the beginning of such sight-threatening conditions as glaucoma or cataract. In most cases, early treatment of eye disease can prevent impairment of vision and even blindness."

The eye is affected by disease and general health of the rest of the body; hence the ophthalmologist diagnoses and treats eye problems as part of the total medical and health care. His treatment may consist of eyeglasses or contact lenses, when necessary, plus orthoptic training, medications, surgery, or any other required scientific therapy. Sometimes an ophthalmologist specializes in surgery to the exclusion of other forms of eye care.

There are about 12,500 practicing ophthalmologists in the United States. Many of them teach; 11 percent conduct research in addition to caring for patients. The ratio of eye physicians to the population is increasing steadily: In 1950 there were only 2.2 per 100,000 population; in 1960 there were 3; in 1970 there were 4; today there are 5 ophthalmologists per 100,000 population and these are predominantly in solo practice. Eye surgery is done by over 90 percent of them, and a major portion of the time ophthalmologists spend in caring for children is devoted to the treatment of crossed eyes.

Education of the ophthalmologist includes four years of college pre-medical training, four years or more of medical school, one year of general medical internship, and three or more years of medical training and experience in eye care hospitals and medical eye clinics (formerly called a medical residency). Ophthalmologists also take postdoctoral courses in the diagnosis and treatment of ocular diseases, application of physiological and optical principles to the prescription of lenses and the correction of aberrations of ocular muscle functions, and in surgery of the eye and its related structures.

Ninety-five percent of practicing eye physicians

in the U.S. are aided in their care of patients by other health professionals such as nurses, medical assistants, optical fitters (including opticians), optical technicians, and others. For example, the ophthalmic medical assistant, also known as the ophthalmic technician or technologist, is an important "right hand" for the ophthalmologist. One to four years of academic and/or on-the-job training in an accredited program at a medical center or an ophthalmologist's office is required. The technologist performs an increasing number of data collection tasks and other technical services required in daily ophthalmology medical practice. The certified ophthalmic medical assistant with evidence of approved continuing education may apply for certification at a higher level. He or she may assist the ophthalmologist in surgery, and in some instances may be a graduate professional nurse.

Another eye care professional using refractive corrections with lenses, the optometrist (pronounced op/TOM/e/trist), has an O.D. degree which represents him or her as a doctor of optometry. The O.D. provides vital primary health care services. For instance, the optometrist examines, diagnoses, and prescribes specific treatment for conditions of the vision system.

Optometrists examine eyes and related structures to determine the presence of vision problems, diseases or other abnormalities. They utilize drugs for diagnostic purposes when permitted by state laws (which are changing throughout the country). By thoroughly evaluating the internal and external structure of the eyes, optometrists can detect systemic and eye diseases that require referral of the patient to other health care practitioners.

The optometrist treats by prescribing and adapting spectacle lenses, contact lenses, or other optical aids and uses visual training/vision therapy to preserve or restore maximum efficiency of vision.

Education of the optometrist includes two to four years of college pre-optometric training and four additional years of specialized professional training at an accredited college of optometry.

In contrast to the other two eye care professionals, the optician (pronounced OP/ti/cian) is not degreed as a doctor. An optician is the technical part of the lens-servicing team. He or she may also be known as a dispensing optician or an ophthalmic dispenser. The optician could be both or either of these designated types of specialists. The dispensing optician makes and fits eyeglasses and/or contact lenses, frames, and other specially fabricated optical devices upon prescription to the intended wearer.

The ophthalmic dispenser both tests people for eyeglasses and also makes and fits them. The ophthalmic dispenser's functions include, but are not limited to, prescription analysis and interpretation, the taking of measurements to determine the size, shape, and specifications of the lenses, frames, contact lenses, or lens forms best suited to the wearer's needs; the preparation and delivery of work orders to laboratory technicians engaged in grinding lenses, and fabricating eyewear; the verification of the quality of finished ophthalmic products; the adjustment of lenses or frames to the intended wearer's face or eyes; and the adjustment, replacement, repair and reproduction of previously prepared ophthalmic lenses, frames, or other specially fabricated ophthalmic devices.

The Politics of the Eyeball

"Eyeball politics" is created by the struggle for potential patient attention among the three eye care professions. Confusion reigns, in particular for the patient, when he or she is forced to determine if eyeglasses and/or contacts should be purchased from the optician who designs, manufactures, and sells lenses and frames or from the optometrist who not only prescribes such lenses but also has them made by prescription and sells them at a profit.

Additionally, the patient must further decide if the optometrist he sees regularly for eyeglass prescriptions is detecting eye health problems. Ophthalmologists say only a medical doctor can do this. Optometrists say they, as O.D.'s, have the training to catch a health problem and refer the patient to an eye surgeon, saving the patient an extra professional visit.

Judith Doctor, M.D., an ophthalmologist practicing in Westport, Connecticut and affiliated with Norwalk Hospital (in Norwalk, Connecticut) says that eye doctors are the sole professionals licensed to use drugs that dilate the pupils, making it easier to spot the early signs of disease. "Only a medical doctor has the training to give a complete medical exam," she added.

Robert Toss, O.D., practicing optometry in Westport, responded that most people who see an optometrist regularly will get the necessary exams to catch eye health problems. He said, "Ninety-six percent of the patients visiting eye professionals have vision, not medical problems, but any possible trouble could be detected by a good optometrist." As an example he referred to a machine in his office that does a sophisticated test for high pressure in the eye, the sign of glaucoma.

Around the country optometrists are lobbying in state legislatures for permission to use drugs that dilate the pupils. Such lobbying for the more medically-oriented effort has angered ophthalmologists, who declare that only those with an M.D. degree should be allowed to administer drugs to eye care patients. They argue that the dilating drugs could trigger a sudden glaucoma attack. Eye physicians are unable to tell when a stimulus might set off an unexpected increase in eye pressure, which may build to dangerous levels, according to Bernard Singer, M.D., chief of the section of ophthalmology at Norwalk Hospital.

If an acute glaucoma attack should strike, it is essential that the patient have a medical doctor on hand to treat the disease, Dr. Singer said. Along with the blinding pain from an acute attack, Dr. Singer stated, "An untreated, undiagnosed acute attack can result in total blindness within twenty-four to forty-eight hours." He added that many such victims will need immediate surgery.

Dr. Ross countered with the statement that the fears of an acute glaucoma attack are overrated. "These kinds of attacks are rare: I don't think a patient should fear getting one when the eye is dilated," Dr. Ross said. He added that the patient could always go to a local hospital with little risk of permanent eye damage.

While optometrists are sparring with ophthalmologists on the right to administer dilating drugs, they are also arguing with opticians about the right to fit contact lenses. There is nothing in most state regulations to prevent an optician from fitting contacts. Many state opticians' licensing examinations include whole sections on contact lenses. Some opticians don't choose to fit contacts and have asked that the part of the test be reserved for those practitioners who choose to go into the field. That way, an optician failing the contact lens portion, but not the eyeglass portion, of the test won't have been deprived from taking a job or opening in an optical shop where eyeglasses are manufactured and sold.

In contrast, optometrists think that opticians do not have the training to fit hard and soft lenses directly on the eye. They say that all opticians should be prevented from doing the detailed work. They suggest that of the soft contact lenses alone, with more than two dozen manufacturers making them in a dizzying variety of shapes, widths, thickness, and materials, more knowledge is needed than available to the less-trained opticians. Some optometrists say, "Opticians don't know which end is up" about contacts. Dr. Ross said, in referring to opticians fitting contact lenses, "It is a violation of the laws of medicine and optometry."

But opticians who do choose to fit contact lenses point to their success with patients. They question the economic motives of the optometrists' efforts to restrict opticians' practices. It's strictly a matter of greed, they declare. An optician who asked not be named said, "An optometrist has a major stake in contacts, but the ophthalmologist can prescribe them too. It hurts the optometrist's business to have the job handled by the ophthalmologist and the optician. It cuts him out." In some cases, the ophthalmologist prescribes the correction and the optician manufactures and sells it. The optometrist is like a barnacle on a boat slowing down the patient's passage to better sight. Opticians agree among themselves that the optometrist appears to be an unnecessary professional addition.

There is more politics mixed up with money and lenses. Ophthalmologists don't usually sell eyeglasses and contact lenses, so they declare themselves above the conflict between eye care professionals and obvious economic interests where lenses are sold. Optometrists point out that this attitude smacks of cover-up.

For instance, optometrists claim they do not push unneeded lenses on patients, even though they sell the products. The ophthalmologists doubt this statement. Optometrists, in turn, claim that some ophthalmologists are not above making a profit on lenses, because they do, in fact, have affiliations with lens stores or opticians. Some eye surgeons have lens dispensing sections right in their offices, and they are not entirely truthful about not profiting from the sale of visual aids.

Finally, the opticians routinely complain that some ophthalmologists and optometrists are slow to furnish prescriptions to other specialists when it becomes clear the patient is going to shop around for the eye care products.

This interprofessional infighting goes on among opticians, optometrists, and ophthalmologists in almost every community in the United States. There is little love about an ongoing power grab at the top rungs of the eye care ladder by optometrists. Optometrists are trying to get maximum mileage out of their training so as to enhance their income by an increased sale of services. With ever-present political resistance from both professions, vision-impaired people become the losers.

Ophthalmologists Open Eyes to Optometrists Power Play

Ophthalmologists once were placed firmly at the top of the eye care "ladder," many rungs above optometrists, dispensing opticians, and all others in the vision field, members of the American Academy of Ophthalmology and Otolaryngology (the

32

study of the ears, nose, and throat) were told at their October 1976 annual meeting. But because eye surgeons were "legislatively asleep," non-physician practitioners, primarily optometrists, have been able to fight for and win increasingly larger shares of the eye care domain.

"Ophthalmology has been overtaken and it is now in the process of being taken over," warned Whitney G. Sampson, M.D., a Houston eye surgeon.

Legislative "battles have not been lost by ophthalmology; they have been forfeited," said Byron H. Demorest, M.D., a Sacramento, California eye physician.

Particularly under the protest of national health insurance, "all practitioners in the ophthalmic field are now scurrying for a position as close to the top of the ladder as possible in order to assure their own professional eminence in the future," Dr. Demorest said.

"The future of ophthalmology rests in the hands, hearts, and minds of our legislators. Supporting and working with local legislators is a high priority item for each doctor who is concerned about the future of his practice and of eye care for his patients. As state and national laws defining the boundaries for eye care practitioners are changed, all of us must carefully monitor such actions," urged Dr. Demorest.

Kenneth J. Myers, O.D., director of optometry for the Veterans Administration (VA), which does not authorize optometrists to use drugs, agreed. Dr. Myers said, "I feel equitable relations can more easily be developed (between optometrists and ophthalmologists) if it is clearly stated VA optometrists will not practice therapeutic medical or surgical eye care . . . VA clinical procedures are now and will continue to be dictated by this basic division of responsibility: Ophthalmology staff definitely diagnoses all medical and surgical ocular conditions and provides any required medical or surgical ocular therapy. Optometry staff provides optometric diagnosis and therapy of vision dysfunction with referral to VA physicians of patients having signs and/or symptoms of ocular disease or injury. It is not our intent to expand the practice of optometry into medical or surgical areas, for we believe these areas are the correct and historically established domain of the physician, and it is best for patient care that optometry and ophthalmology continue centered in their respective disciplines."

Calling himself "middle of the road" in the ophthalmology-optometry dispute, David M. Worthen, M.D., head of ophthalmology at the

University of California, San Diego, said, "In my opinion, the present optometrist is overtrained for what he can do, yet doesn't receive an education of high enough quality to allow him to give complete care." The prescribing of medicines, especially, he said, "just like the performance of surgery, must be founded on a broad-based medical curriculum," which optometrists generally do not receive.

"To allow any health care provider to prescribe therapeutic medicines or operate on the basis of limited classroom experience is the practice of medicine without a license and should be stopped, regardless of legislative changes. In my opinion, such erosion will lower the quality of medical care in all areas," said Dr. Worthen.

Of course, another area of dispute exists between optometrists and ophthalmologists—the area of eye surgery for refractive problems. Optometrists don't perform surgery but just prescribe corrective lenses. Ophthalmologists do both. Optometrists have been accused of discouraging people from engaging in surgical corrections strictly because surgery competes directly with the prescribing of lenses by them. Such discouragement of people from undertaking permanent correction by operative means to eliminate eyeglasses and contacts is considered unethical and an exploitation of trusting individuals.

Ophthalmologists additionally suggest that optometrists sometimes overprescribe eyeglasses for minimal refractive errors. They say that the total cost of examination and glasses by an optometrist could exceed that given by an ophthalmologist. If lessened expense is the object, refractive care delivered by trained ophthalmic assistants working under the direct supervision of ophthalmologists costs less and supposedly gives the patient equivalent care.

Frequently a patient with a serious eye problem first consults an optometrist for examination. Many individuals have been conditioned to believe that lenses are able to accommodate most eye difficulties, which is untrue. Finding that the problem consists of more than the simple need for a lens correction, the honest optometrist will likely refer his visitor on to the patient's physician for a reexamination. With a serious eye disorder present, the average family doctor probably won't feel qualified to treat it. Finally the patient is referred, in turn, to the ophthalmologist who should have been consulted in the first place.

This situation, or a similar set of circumstances, is what may bring someone to seek eye surgery such as radial keratotomy (RK) or another of the operative refractive corrections. Indeed, controversy prevails within the ophthalmology profession about these various refractive surgeries which we will be describing in later in this book.

The Ophthalmic Controversy Over Radial Keratotomy

Several years ago in Marietta, Georgia, 32 year-old nearsighted Alfred Gresham, an engineer, underwent RK for his right eye. Gresham was ready to have his left eye operated on for curing his nearsightedness, but the man found himself caught in the middle of a small but polite war between his eye surgeon and the Georgia Ophthalmological Society. This professional body, warning of the danger of possible delayed side-effects from the RK operation which is spreading rapidly in the United States and overseas, persuaded Georgia state hospitals to temporarily ban the procedure in their operating rooms. Studies which by now have convinced most ophthalmologists that RK is a valid, safe, effective operation for permanent correction of nearsightedness had not yet been carried out.

Gresham told us then that he was "mad as hell" about the "medical politics" which might have prevented the operation on his right eye until the Georgia Ophthalmological Society conducted what could be a multi-year investigation "to determine the procedure's effectiveness and safety." This is still sometimes found to be the attitude expressed by some traditionalists in ophthalmology who don't have training in performing radial keratotomy or the other breakthrough methods of high-tech vision improvement.

Until the fall of 1984, with presentation of the Prospective Evaluation of Radial Keratotomy, (PERK) study, the American Association of Ophthalmology (AAO) considered the RK procedure investigational rather than experimental. Surgeons who supported the procedure—numbering among them some of the nation's most distinguished professors and eye surgeons, including one former president of the AAO - agreed that the answers won't be all put together about side effects until patients have reached the post-surgery mark twenty years from now. But, based on experience with more complex corneal surgery and with accidental corneal injury, they foresee no serious problems ahead.

Nevertheless, controversy in ophthalmology about refractive surgery continues. It is rife and disagreements are heated among eye physicians when it comes to RK. For example, Long Island, New York ophthalmologist Norman O. Stahl, M.D., was banned from doing RK at his hospital. He could not practice the procedure there and warnings came down from the administration office that he might be thrown out if he continued to try. Dr.

Stahl responded by setting up a surgical suite in his private office. No one could stop him from performing the dozens of myopia-correction procedures there.

Since Dr. Stahl took this step, in fact, in-office surgery - called "office-based surgery" - not only for eyes but for a host of other body problems has become rather common. An entirely new medical industry to cut the cost of medical care by eliminating hospital expenses has arisen with the new office-based surgery.

At least four professional groups have been pooling data about RK in order to make some judgments about its safety and effectiveness. They include the National Institute of Health-funded multi-university study headed by George Waring, M.D. of Atlanta, Georgia; the National Refractive Keratotomy study group under the direction of Leo Bores, M.D. of White Plains, New York. Additionally, the National Advisory Eye Council has put out a call to all patients who have undergone RK and to all optometrists who have refracted the eyes of such patients to report their observations.

The National Advisory Eye Council is the principal advisory group to the National Eye Institute. In order to discharge its responsibilities to the American public and to the scientific and health care community, the Council has acquired as much information as possible about the safety of RK on humans. The Council has urged people to share whatever information they may possess about eye problems that have resulted from this surgical procedure.

In addition to complications of the cooperative effort itself, the Council members were looking for any secondary problems, such as ocular rupture or perforation. Ronald G. Geller, Ph.D., Executive Secretary of the National Eye Institute, advises interested physicians and patients about his survey results. They indicate that no such problems or side effects exist for recipients of radial keratotomy.

Some opponents of RK have attempted to suppress the availability of the operation. They have tried to institute a moratorium on the procedure. They also encouraged health insurance companies not to reimburse patients who ordinarily would be covered for financial outlays.

Chapter 3

Lenses To Protect And Correct The Eyes

Bernice Pherigo of Columbus, Indiana, blind for forty-two years, could see again because of an unusual device like a telescope that passes images through a hole in her eyelid to her retina. The device is a Teflon disc in an optical cylinder - a lens developed in the early 1970s by Hernando Cardona, M.D., an ophthalmologist on the staff of Columbia University.

In the fall of 1977, the patient, who was then sixty-five years old, had the lens implanted into her right eye by Frank Polak, M.D. of the Florida Health Center's Eye Clinic in Gainesville, Florida. The woman had lost her vision in both eyes when she was in her twenties because of a disease called ocular pemphigus. The diesase causes blisters and scars on the outer surface of the eye. In Miss Pherigo's case, the scar tissue was removed several

41

times in surgery but continued to grow back. Her vision deteriorated to the point where she could only distinguish between light and darkness.

All that is changed today, for the combination of eye surgery and corrective lenses has Miss Pherigo seeing again. Over the past few years the woman has been getting acquainted with a technological phenomenon that passed her by in her forty-year period without sight. Now she's watching movements on a television screen. There are worlds of small joys such as colors, and the look of furniture in her apartment that she has been experiencing. The vision in Bernice Pherigo's right eye is about 20/40 now. She can read large-print magazines and newspapers, and eyeglasses have been added to improve her vision of faraway objects.

Working like a fixed-focus camera, the lens in Bernice's eye receives light and transmits it to the eye's retina, where the image is recorded. The patient's upper and lower eyelids have been permanently stitched together and the lens protrudes through a hole in the eyelid. There is no peripheral vision, but Miss Pherigo can move the cylinder with muscles that normally open and close the eyelid.

Cases such as this of Bernice Pherigo are highly dramatic applications of lenses used to restore sight. Those few blind people who have normal retinas and whose corneal damage cannot be repaired by cornea transplant can benefit from a lens implantation. Other people not requiring such dramatic restoration wear ordinary eyeglasses to preserve and enhance the vision that they possess.

The purchase of a new, or first pair of eyeglasses is ofter a mystifying experience for the most of the multimillions who wear corrective lenses. Indeed, there is more to acquiring spectacles then selecting appealing frames.

"Shop around, compare prices, and know what services to expect both from you ophthalmologist who prescribes the glasses and from the optician who will make them," suggested Alfonse A. Cinotti, M.D., former president of the American Association of Ophthalmology. "At the time of your eye examination, if glasses are required, your ophthalmologist should provide you with a copy of your eyeglass prescription at no additional charge. This is unquestionably the right of every patient. With the prescription in hand you may choose to visit a local optician, or if your ophthalmologist dispenses glasses, you may choose to purchase them from him or her."

"If the prescription is properly filled, your glasses should provide you with vision which you feel is adequate," said Burton M. Krimmer, M.D., a Chicago ophthalmologist. "A correct prescription alone does not insure that your glasses will feel comfortable on your face. You should check to make sure that the frames sit well upon your face. If the fit is wrong, they might slip off your nose and create a vision distortion and general feeling of discomfort. Though sometimes fashionable, very large frames, or lenses can cause problems," Dr. Krimmer added. "It is advisable to select a small frame and a small lens for the higher prescriptions required to correct vision problems like strong astigmatism, or severe nearsightedness or farsightedness. This is because the smaller size assures the patient a more accurately ground lens."

If visual discomfort persists after wearing the new eyeglasses for several days, they should be checked for accuracy by a trained member of the ophthalmologist's staff. The eye doctor will want to verify that the optician has properly filled the prescription. He will determine if the spectacles themselves are centered, and if the pupil distance, the optical center of near and far vision, has been correctly measured. Also checked will be the base curvature of the lens (the curvature of the glass) and that it has been accurately ground. The ophthalmologist will comfirm that the front and the back of the lens is correct. Without this final checkup, a visual annoyance could develop if an inaccuracy exists.

Comsumer awareness should not be disregarded once you have your new eyeglasses at home. Pulling the spectacles off the face with one hand may destroy their alignment. Remove them with both hands, one on each side. This is an important point which should be emphasized when young children first receive eyeglasses.

"Care for your frames and lenses the way you would care for a fine instrument," suggested Dr. Krimmer. "Never lay your glasses down when you are not using them. Put them away in a good storage case."

A proper storage case should have a soft lining which will not abrade the lenses. And it should have a supportive outer shell which will not easily be crushed and may thus protect your eyeglasses. Never store spectacles in an unlined leather case. Leather scratches and may damage the lenses. Don't store your eyeglasses in a case which is too restrictive inasmuch as most frames are made of plastic, and this could compress them out of shape.

If your vision does require a new lens prescription, it is possible that your old frames may not be satisfactory. The fitter should be aware of this situation and tell you whether or not the old frames are serviceable and if continued use is economical. "There is absolutely no truth to the myth that you should have your eyeglasses checked each year,"

45

said Dr. Krimmer. "The eye doctor will usually advise an appropriate interval between exams, depending upon your individual needs."

"Glasses have nothing to do with the health of the eyes," confirmed Paul R. Lichter, M.D., a University of Michigan ophthalmologist. "Having them checked annually is somewhat like going to the shoe store each year to see if you need new shoes. So long as a person is pleased with the vision he has with his present eyeglasses, there is little reason to check for a change."

You should also be aware of other myths. "The way light enters the eye is, to many people, a mysterious event." Therefore, Dr. Lichter continued, "there is a belief that if light doesn't enter the eye properly something bad will happen. Sitting too close to a television set, reading a dim light, holding a book too close, or wearing someone else's glasses, all evoke a feeling of danger in the public's mind. In fact, the eye deals with light regardless of how it enters the eye. Whether the light is dim, or the rays are bent in one way or another, the eye will still perform its function. Nothing unhealthy can result from this."

Another thing the eye specialist reported is that speaking of eyeglasses which are "too strong" is simply a misnomer. What patients usually mean is that their eyeglasses are uncomfortable. This discomfort may be annoying, but it will not cause harm to the eyes.

How Best to Utilize Sunglasses

Have practical considerations in mind when you choose a pair of sunglasses. Read the label when examining the light transmission factor. Eyeglasses for the sun should transmit no more than 30 percent of the light; select those that transmit only 10 to 15 percent for use on the beach, water, or snow. Make sure they're dark enough so that you can't see your eyes through them when looking in a mirror. Polarizing lenses do help reduce glare during boating or driving, but for intense glare, mirrored lenses are best.

Portions of the eyes absorb the rays of the sun even without our knowing it. The infrared—or heat—waves, for example, are absorbed partly by the cornea and partly by the lens, but a surprisingly large amount reach the retina.

The cornea is that main recipient of almost all the ultraviolet rays. What the cornea doesn't absorb, the lens of the eye will. Because of this, prolonged exposure to ultraviolet rays will be mainly felt on the cornea, which may blister and cause extreme pain.

Gradient density lenses, those which are darker at the top of the glass than near the bottom, originally were developed for pilots. When flying, the pilot needs the sunglasses for the bright sky, but must also be able to read the dials in the dim cockpit. The bottom portion of the sunglasses, therefore, is perfect for the in-cabin instruments view.

But these glasses are not really suited to the average person's needs. Usually, just as much harmful glare is bouncing up from the sidewalks, beaches and water as is from the sky. Therefore, the lighter lower half of the lenses is virtually useless as protection.

Phototropic lenses, sometimes called photo-chromic, adjust to the light intensity of the environment. They remain clear when there is little or no sunlight and turn darker with increasing brightness. They are convenient especially for those who must where corrective eyeglasses constantly. It eliminates the need to by a second prescription pair just for sunglasses.

Some eye experts warn that one is not receiving enough protection from infrared rays. The range of phototropic lenses is not sufficient, they say, to change from completely clear to completely dark. Moreover, the lenses will retain a smoky pink hue—even at night—following repeated exposure to ultraviolet rays.

Even now, the sunglasses do not darken enough, claim some professionals, to protect the eyes from glare that one would need while on a beach. Using phototropic lenses during an extended stay by the ocean may, in fact, result in degraded night vision.

Because of the questionable protection they provide, phototropic lenses are not recommended for use by older adults. who are particularly sensitive to eye damage.

Plastic polarized sunglasses are advertised for their ability to reduce the glare reflected off flat surfaces. But they lack the infrared filtering system. In fact, all plastic sunglasses lack this important ability. In cool climates, however, a good pair of plastic sunglasses may be sufficient. They are inadequate, though, in the areas which experience hotter summers.

So what type of sunglasses should you wear? The best contain properly-made dark gray glass lenses. Their "smoke" tint allows one to see colors in the most natural way. The lenses' effectiveness depends upon the chemical ingredient added to it to produce the color.

Second best are green glass lenses followed by shades of brown in the glass. The "fashion sunglasses" in shades of blues and yellows offer no protection, regardless of how dark the lenses are. Yellow lenses, though, are helpful to hunters, pilots and athletes who spend a great deal of time outside. This color will improve visibility on a hazy or cloudy day.

Avoid wearing sunglasses indoors or after dark; it's a bad habit which may lead to night vision impairment. In a tanning hut or under an ultraviolet lamp, substitute sun goggles for sunglasses so as to not bring on damage to the sensitive areas of the eyes. You can burn them.

Burned eyes, indeed, are the most common summer eye problem, reported Robert J. Crossen, M.D., a former trustee of the American Association of Ophthalmology. There is growing evidence the burn is caused at least, partially, by infrared rays. Ultraviolet rays will damage the cornea, too, a problem that may not reveal itself until the next day. Then you may awaken from sleep with searing pain and a feeling of sand grains in the eyes. Sometimes the cornea could be so scarred, vision is impaired.

Night vision may be reduced by too much exposure to the sun. You might not be able to drive home safely after staying the bright sun for a prolonged period. Those who have their occupations on the sea, in the snow, or on desert sands, could develop cataracts from an excess exposure to sunlight accumulated over the years.

The impact-resistant lenses required by the U.S. Food and Drug Administration (FDA) in all eyeglasses and sunglasses supplied to the public after December 31, 1971 are not all shatter-proof or break-proof. Although impact-resistant lenses afford greater protection than previously provided, they don't furnish an unbreakable shield against eye injury. The FDA regulation only asks that eyeglasses and sunglasses have heat-treated glass lenses, plastic lenses, laminated glass lenses or glass lenses made impact-resistant by other means. They must be capable of withstanding an impact test in which a 5/8 inch steel ball is dropped on the lens from a height of 50 inches. And the regulation does not cover contact lenses.

COMPARATIVE LIGHT TRANSMISSION FACTORS
of SUNGLASSES

Color		Ultra Violet	Visible Light	Infra Red	Uses
CLEAR		7%	7%	7%	
PINK	Light	95%	10%	10%	Cuts glare from artificial lights.
	Medium	95%	15-20%	10%	
	Dark	95%	45-50%	15%	
BLUE	Light	95%	10%	5%	Cuts glare from artificial lights.
	Medium	95%	25%	10%	Cosmetic NOT for sun.
	Dark	95%	70%	12%	
GREEN	Light	75%	15%	55%	Cataract glasses.
	Medium	99%	35%	98%	Cool climate glasses.
	Dark	99%	70%	99%	Good sunglasses.
BROWN	Light	95%	20-40%	35%	Cool climate sunglasses and cuts through blue haze.
	Medium	97%	65%	50%	Sunglasses.
	Dark	99%	80%	80%	
GRAY	Light	95%	20-40%	60%	Cool climate sunglasses or not to sensitive to light.
	Medium	98%	80%	80%	
YELLOW		95%	15%	10%	Increase visibility in haze and fog.
PHOTO-TROPIC	Light	85%	15-20%	15%	General wear and winter sports sunglasses in cool climate
	Dark	85%	20-70%	15%	

Contact Lens Advances

Technology is creating contact lenses for reasons other than to improve one's nearsightedness. Listed below are three new advances in contact lenses.

Bandage Lenses. Used to protect the eyes of people experiencing cornea problems, these lenses are larger and thinner than a regular contact lens. This "bandage" reduces the pain the eyelid causes as it moves across the tender eye, explains Dr. Wayne Cannon, chair of the contact lens division of the American Optometic Association. It also helps to prevent infections in the eye.

Medicated Contacts. These are still in the experimental stage, but look promising. They were created to treat infections that are difficult to eradicate with eyedrops. The contact lens stores the medication and gradually releases it into the eye. Dr. Cannon explains that the concentration of the medication remains much higher over a longer period of time, which gives it a higher cure rate than eyedrops.

Lens to Correct Color Blindness. These soft contacts are not yet approved by the Food and Drug Administration. The red lens, according to Dr. Cannon, helps people with certain types of color blindness to discriminate colors better. While red lenses have been available on eyeglasses and hard contacts for some time, they were seldom used beause of the unattractive red tint. With the soft lenses, the tint is less noticeable, according to the contact's developers.

53

Pros and Cons of Contact Lens

What is transparent, plastic, about the size of your pinky fingernail, and able to stop traffic when it is lost? Over the last four decades the contact lens has been employed more and more as a substitute for eyeglasses. People with impaired vision often use contacts to conceal their need for visual aid.

Leonardo da Vinci is credited with the original concept of lenses directly in contact with the eyeballs. But his idea lay dormant for several centuries until a Swiss eye doctor prescribed a glass shell in 1887 for a patient with a cancerous eyelid.

Today, refinements and innovations have come swiftly on the heels of each other to render the contact lens of a decade ago obsolete. Recently a lens made by the Dow Corning Corporation has received the approval of the FDA to market the first silicone-based lens for extended wear by cataract patients. The extended wear lens, like others approved by the Federal agency, can be worn for up to a month.

Silicone is a combination of inorganic silicon, the basic component in glass, and organic (carbon-based) materials. Researchers have long believed the material would be ideal for use in contact lenses because oxygen passes freely through it.

54

The eye needs to receive oxygen from the air because the portion covered by the typical contact lens has no blood circulating through it, and the amount of oxygen getting through the lens is a key factor in safety and comfort.

Bausch & Lomb, Inc. and Wesley-Jessen, Inc., a subsidiary of the Schering-Plough Corporation, introduced their 13.5-millimeter bifocal contact lenses in the fall of 1981 but without FDA approval. In January 1982, the agency ordered sales halted until the products could be tested. The FDA says a company trying to sell bifocal soft contact lenses must monitor their use by at least one hundred patients for at least three months to show that they are safe and effective.

Unlike monofocal contact lenses, which are made of round hard glass with equally distributed corrective power, the bifocal lenses are made of soft plastic with separate power ranges. The top of Wesley-Jessen's almost square-shaped bifocal lens, for instance, is designed for distant sight while the bottom has corrective power for reading, or near vision. These soft bifocals are produced with the same manufacturing process as the monofocals, using the same material and employing the same design. The FDA disagrees with their use, and even in 1984, has refused to allow the marketing of soft contact bifocals.

The Ciba-Geigy Corporation and American Hydron, a subsidiary of the National Patent Development Corporation, are waiting to see what will happen. They are also ready to introduce soft bifocal contact lenses. It is estimated that 35 million Americans are potential customers for such lenses, which could mean a market totalling about $250 million.

But, like so many other advances of medicine, contact lenses are a mixed blessing. While they grant freedom from annoyances and limitations of spectacles and in many cases provide superior vision, they can threaten the very thing they are meant to help. If improperly fitted or mishandled, contact lenses can harm your eyesight.

The technical difference between spectacles and contact lenses, said the director of the glaucoma and contact lens services at St. Vincent's Hospital and Medical Center of New York, G. Peter Halberg, M.D., who was president of the Contact Lens Association of Ophthalmologists, is that "Glasses alter the rays to accommodate the defect before they reach the eye. The contact lenses unite the rays inside the eye where they are supposed to unite by actually putting a new surface on the cornea. They are a prosthesis floating on a layer of tears."

However, Dr. Halberg added, "The difference

between perfection and disaster is a hairline. On a long term basis, an ill-fitting contact lens can deform the eye."

To find the specialist who won't cross the hairline, Morton D. Sarver, O.D., professor of optometry at the University of California School of Optometry at Berkeley and chief of the contact lens service there, said, "The concerned consumer must seek the services of a fitter who is familiar with and has access to all the different lenses available. Consult with people who have been well fitted, get a recommendation from a professional society, call an university with an optometrical or ophthalmological department. The question is similar to asking how to find the best surgeon to perform an appendectomy."

Of the basic types of lenses - hard, soft, gas-permeable, silicon - differences among them primarily are in the ways they allow the eye to obtain the nutrients that keep it healthy. As mentioned, because the surface of the cornea does not contain blood vessels, it is dependent upon the flow of tears to obtain oxygen and release carbon dioxide. That is a problem with the element silicon. It is hydrophobic, or "water-hating." Such a characteristic has made it impossible, until now, to get the lenses to ride comfortably on a thin film of tears instead of clinging to the eye.

The soft lens is hydrophilic, or "water-loving," it absorbs water, so it keeps the eye bathed in fluid. Oxygen reaches the cornea in two ways; by direct passage through the lens and from the tear fluid under the lens. The soft lens fits flush against the cornea, assuming whatever shape it has. Such a lens is inappropriate for a person with an irregular cornea, though newer lenses have been developed to oversome this limitation.

More comfortable than hard lenses, soft lenses require little adjustment. They can be worn for a full twenty-four hours just a few days after first acquiring them. Athletes prefer soft lenses because they are less likely than hard lenses to pop out of the eye and are better at keeping out dust and soot. But they cost more initially and during routine care they are more likely to tear and become clouded. A clouded lens, which happens about every two years, must be replaced. Permanent lens clouding and serious eye infection can occur from poor daily cleaning (done with a chemical solution or by boiling).

If they are permitted to dry out, soft lenses become hard but the softness can be restored by placing them in a special salt water solution. Keep in mind that they absorb not only water, but other solutions as well. Do not use eye drops while wearing them. Also don't clean them with the regular solutions used in the care of hard contact lenses. Don't place them in any liquid except the solutions your doctor will instruct you to use. Soft lenses should be removed before swimming or when you are in the presence of irritating vapors.

The person with a significant degree of astigmatism or small degree of farsightedness will not get the required correction from soft contact lenses. The decision concerning suitability must be made individually for each potential wearer.

Among new lens wearers, soft contacts are favored two to one over hard contact lenses. Still, hard contacts do provide superior visual correction. They are less expensive, more durable, require minimal care - daily removal and simple cleaning - may be polished to remove scratches, and reground to adjust to small changes in the eyes. But hard contacts require a protracted break-in period. They are difficult to get used to and must gradually be worn for hours at first and then only up to eighteen hours at a time. If you stop wearing them for a few days, you must repeat the gradual breaking-in process. Rushing the adjustment can lead to painful eye inflammations.

Made of a special hard plastic, as well, the gas-permeable contact lens is more expensive than the standard polymethyl methacrylate hard contact. It lets through oxygen and carbon dioxide, enabling the cornea to "breathe." The gas-permeable lens seems more comfortable to most people. They adapt to it faster than the regular hard lens. If you need the visual correction offered by a hard lens but cannot tolerate the conventional type, the gas-permeable one is probably preferable.

The American Association of Ophthalmology warns that there are certain conditions which make the wearing of contact lenses inadvisable. Examples are chronic inflammation, infection, or allergy affecting the eyes. Some persons suffer from chronic dryness of the eyes due to a deficiency of tears; this may make it impossible for them to tolerate contact lenses. A person who cannot manipulate small objects with ease because of arthritis or a tumor affecting the hands is also not a proper candidate for contact lenses. There may be some transient discomfort during the intitial period of adjusting oneself to contacts. You may experience discomfort if a bit of foreign matter gets into your eye and lodges behind the lens.

At the beginning of this subsection on contacts we suggested that loss of a contact lens could stop traffic. In fact, if your lens should become dislodged or lost while you are driving, a serious hazard would result. Persons who wear contacts and do a lot of driving are advised to carry a spare set of lenses.

If you have an illness which might cause you to lose consciousness at times, as with diabetes or epilepsy, you should wear a medical information bracelet which, alone with other vital information, records the fact that you are wearing contact lenses. In an emergency, the person providing medical care would be alerted to remove the lenses. Hard contacts should never be worn during sleep. The natural blink reflex keeps fluid circulating under the lens; this is necessary to the metabolism of the cornea. Normal fluid circulation ceases when the patient sleeps with his contact lenses in place.

Finally, here are some miscellaneous tips for contact lens wearers:

1. Wait a half hour after awakening before inserting your lenses to give your sleep-swollen corneas a chance to return to normal.

2. A short nap with lenses in place won't be harmful, but remember not to go to bed for the night with your contacts on.

3. Insert lenses prior to putting on face or eye makeup. Water-soluble eye makeup is best for lens wearers.

4. Wash your hands before putting in a lens to avoid introducing irritating substances into the eyes.

5. Never touch the inner surface of the lens which rests against the cornea.

61

6. If you must use aerosol deodorants and hair sprays (and for the sake of the environment it's recommended that you do not), apply them before installing your contact lenses.

7. Have new lenses rechecked after ten days and again in a month to be sure they are not damaging the eyes. Repeat such examinations once a year.

8. See an ophthalmologist if you develop lasting irritation, redness, pain, blurred vision, or any other eye abnormality, whether or not directly connected to your wearing of contact lenses.

Be Cautious of Orthokeratology

The American Association of Ophthalmology (AAO) also warns about a possibly harmful system of tight-fitting contact lenses used to reshape the eye by someone hoping to eliminate the use of surgery, eyeglasses, or contact lenses forever.

Orthokeratology is a technique that appeals to the vanity of the nearsighted person who has worn spectacles all his life. Orthokeratology is untested, costly, and may in the long run prove detrimental, says the AAO. With the little formal research available on the technique, "it seems to be more a gimmick than anything else," cautioned former president Dr. Alfonse Cinotti.

The gimmick is a promise of adequate vision without the burden of visual aids, a promise that appeals to myopic people who should have eye correction with lenses or surgery but refuse. Myopics have the eyeball misshapened; it is too long or too steep. Therefore, light that enters the eye has to travel a greater distance to hit the retina than it travels in the normal eye. Light and the image it carries falls short of focusing on the retina, causing myopia, which is an inability to see things at a distance.

In an attempt to correct this nearsightedness through the technique of orthokeratology, a series of increasingly tighter fitting contact lenses are used over a period of time in an effort to reshape the cornea. Supposedly, the tight fitting lenses flatten this soft tissue which covers the eye, making the eye shorter, so light focuses where it should, directly on the retina.

"But there is not enough scientific information about orthokeratology to say whether it's useful or worthless," said Dr. Burton Krimmer, the ophthalmologist from Chicago whom we also cited earlier. "So far there have been no control studies and most of the information is anecdotal - word of mouth." Dr. Krimmer added that the dangers of orthokeratology appear to be greater than any values it has to offer.

"When contact lenses are too tight they disturb the transfer of gases in and out of the cornea. This disturbance can cause the cornea to become cloudy or even ulcerated - painful and harmful conditions," Dr. Krimmer continued.

Corneal ulcers, which are similar to bedsores that occur when there has been pressure too long on one spot, are infections that can lead to the loss of the eye, explained Philip Hessburg, M.D., an ophthalmologist from Michigan. Dr. Hessburg charged that the underlying theory of orthokeratology, the permanent change of soft tissue with a temporary device, appeared to be unsound.

"To my knowledge, there is no evidence to show that we can permanently alter the shape of any soft tissue," he said, "if we could do so, we could correct protruding ears by taping them down at night or lift up the jowly chin with slings one sees sold near the backs of ladies magazines. We could destroy the bra and girdle industry if the use of their garments permanently molded soft tissue," Dr. Hessburg assured.

Why then would anyone resort to orthokeratology? It has worked in some people who are slightly myopic, the AAO acknowledges. But these myopics probably don't even have to wear regular contact lenses because their nearsightedness is so slight.

Orthokeratology also produces a temporary change in vision after a while. This might appeal to the person who wants to pass a job interview without any optical device, suggested Dr. Krimmer. He added, though, that people who are required to have perfect eyesight for their jobs, like pilots, may put themselves as well as other people in danger.

Dr. Cinotti says because of the cost factor alone, he would not recommend orthokeratology to his patients. "If you have a high refractive error, orthokeratology will make little difference," he points out. "There is no reason you should not use ordinary contact lenses that cost less. And there is no great advantage with orthokeratology for people where the error is not so high. Such people can go through the procedure at a cost of perhaps $2,000, experience slight change in vision, and still have to buy contact lenses and wear them as retainers at night. I tell people - keep your present lenses with which you're comfortable and save money."

Eye Protection at Home, at Work, and in Sports

Numerous accidents and substances can negatively affect the eye. Heavily chlorinated pools can cause a mild chemical burn of the cornea, resulting in scratchy feelings in the eyes. Eye infections come from public swimming pools and ponds which may be prevented by wearing watertight swim goggles or face masks.

Next to cataract, eye injury is the most common cause of visual impairment in the United States today, warns the National Society to Prevent Blindness (NSPB). Virginia S. Boyce, executive director of the 75-year-old voluntary sight-saving organization, points out that a million Americans are permanent causalities of accidental eye damage, most of it occurring in ordinary everyday activities. Forty-five percent of vision-impairing injuries occur around the home.

"Accidents will happen," Mrs. Boyce said. "These often can't be prevented." Ammonia, lye, and other harsh chemicals found in household cleaners and garden sprays are particularly damaging to the eye, resulting in injury, burns - even blindness. She recommends that you read package labels and instructions thoroughly before using such products. Many give specific directions, and ignoring them can result in injuries. Use special caution with pressurized spray cans. Be sure the spray nozzle is directed away from you. Spray cans make tempting toys, so be sure to keep them well out of reach of children.

Wood slivers, rocks, metal pieces, and other particles thrown off by hand tools and power equipment like drills, welding equipment, and chain saws also cause serious eye damage. Lawnmowers, frequently a cause of eye injuries, can hurl a stone at high speed into your eye or some unsuspecting bystander. Keep young children away when you're mowing. Be sure that all tools and machinery are kept in good repair.

In 1983, 12,028 Americans were treated in hospital emergency rooms for injuries from fireworks, almost one-third more than the total reported for 1982. Nearly 15 percent of those injuries were to the eye, reports Mrs. Boyce's National Society to Prevent Blindness. "Since there is no way to estimate how many were treated in doctor's offices, at home, or by direct hospital admission, this figure is only a fraction of actual injuries," said the NSPB executive director. "Sparklers, firecrackers, bottlerockets, M-80's - these and all fireworks endanger the eyes. They may seem harmless, but even sparklers burn at heat exceeding 1500 degrees F."

For many years the Society has urged that fireworks be limited to licensed public displays. Although this is law in twenty-eight states, bootleg fireworks are still sold regularly on street corners and in many stores. The struggle goes on to save eyesight even though people do things to themselves. "Those nineteen and under suffered nearly two-thirds of the injuries last year," Mrs. Boyce noted, adding that "the victims are frequently innocent bystanders. Keep your children away from all fireworks and from anyone who uses them. They may look like fun to youngsters, but fireworks are explosives that can cause injuries, even blindness".

Three days after Independence Day 1984, on July 7th, it was announced by the media that 8,490 people, mostly children, were treated for injuries from the use of fireworks on the Fourth of July alone. Fireworks should be banned for private use and only shown in displays by authorized agencies hiring professionals to handle them.

Incidentally, Mrs. Boyce advises that if getting to the eye doctor is something you keep putting off, you can perform some simple eye tests at home with a kit from the NSPB. The Home Eye Test for Adults checks distance vision, near vision, and whether or not you have macular degeneration, a disorder of the eye anterior. If you fail any of the tests, you should visit an eye specialist. The kit costs $1 from the National Society to Prevent Blindness, 70 Madison Avenue, New York City, New York, 10016; Telephone, (212) 684-3505.

Tips For Treating Eye Injuries

Very few of us survived childhood without receiving at least one black eye. We all remember relatives exclaiming, almost in admiration, "What a shiner!"

Usually, a black eye is nothing more than bruised tissue around the eye. There are times, though, when it can cause more serious damage. If, after receiving an eye injury, you experience double vision or other problems with your sight, contact your ophthalmologist immediately.

Generally speaking, if an eye injury hurts more when you blink, professional help should be sought. It is best to patch the eye in the interval between recognizing the seriousness of the condition and seeing a doctor.

The following is one of the best methods for patching an eye:

* Gently place a cottonball or two over the closed, injured eye.

* Attach strips of tape to the forehead and cheeks in an overlapping manner. This prevents light from entering the eye.

* Have the person open his good eye. He should not be able to see any light through the patched eye.

The most common eye injury is the entrance of a foreign object between the eyeball and the lid. At one time or another everyone experiences this. Your eye will automatically tear, which cleanses the area and

---

Tips For Treating Eye Injuries (con't)

usually flushes the object out. Any situation more serious than this should be examined by a doctor.

There are those times when you need to examine a peron's eye to determine whether an object is in it. Carefully follow these instructions:

1. Have the person lay on his back in a dark room. Ask him to look at the ceiling.

2. Carefully look under the person's lower eyelid by gently pulling down on the skin beneath the lid. In this manner, you can easily see inside the sac, with the aid of a flashlight.

3. Have the person look at his feet, still laying on his back. Gently take the upper eyelid lashes with your left hand while gently depressing the skin of his upper lid downward. This will turn the eyelid inside out and effectively allow you to examine the eye.

4. Should you discover an object, take a very thin wisp of cotton and attempt to dislodge it and lift it up. If this is not possible, run water over the eye from a small glass or eye cup. This usually will wash the object out into the eye, where his blinking will eventually lodge it into one of the corners of the eye.

Employing Safety Goggles

A young racquetball player from Peoria, Illinois, Marcie O'Shaunessy, had her eye cut open when her opponent's racquet struck and mashed her eyeglasses. Luckily for Marcie, surgical repair saved her vision. Now she is back playing racquetball, but she always makes sure to wear special impact-resistant safety goggles ground to her prescription.

Such an accident to one or both eyes is not uncommon in sports activities, since Americans are exceedingly competitive and exercise conscious. Each year, over 35,000 people suffer eye injuries that impair vision. Ophthalmologists have noted an alarming increase in eye traumas, especially during these summer months. Tennis, hockey, cycling, basketball, football, and other recreational activities are the culprits. Yet, the National Society to Prevent Blindness has indicated that ninety percent of all eye injuries can be prevented with proper safety equipment or, as a result of accidents happening out of uncorrected visual impairment, with refractive surgery or external visual aids.

Sports eye protectors, which are goggle-type molded eyeguards, with or without corrected lenses are most useful. They can be made with one's prescription built in. A full lens is recommended for badminton, cycling, yard work, woodworking, and other do-it-yourself ventures. They may be acquired from eye doctors, sporting good stores, racquet clubs, and opticians.

71

Ophthalmologist Paul F. Vinger, M.D. of Lexington, Massachusetts suggested that the best protection is offered by optical quality polycarbonate lenses, which can withstand very high-intensity blows. One such product, Action Eyes, is made by Bausch & Lomb. Another is called Pro-tek Gargoyles and are injection-molded, wraparound, lightweight, shatterproof eye protectors with clear or sunglass tint, useful for skiing and cycling as well as racquet sports.

Dr. Vinger also recommended that safety goggles should be worn when trimming shrubs, using a power mower or workshop tools, or spraying paint or pesticides. Goggles can protect your eyes from the irritating smoke of a barbecue.

With some non-contact sports such as track and bicycling you're able to participate wearing eyeglasses or contact lenses. With others such as swimming, diving, gymnastics, karate, judo, and more, corrective lenses are impossible to use. Surely permanent refractive correction with the newest medical breakthrough, which the author has named "high-tech vision," is of vital importance to those sportspersons who are nearsighted, farsighted, or have astigmatism but can't use external aids for their vision.

Besides the newly introduced refractive surgical techniques, contacts and spectacles have been the two main forms of correction for difficulties with one's cornea. Special lenses may have been recommended for your particular sport or occupation. For example, a golfer could order special eyeglasses that possess built-in corrections for addressing the ball and another lens change for watching the ball wing its way down the fairway. Target and trap shooters might wear specially made eyeglasses for seeing their gun sights and a second correction for visualizing the targets afar. These types of external aids are called functional eyeglasses. They can be tailored for the individualized seeing requirements of your sport or hobby.

But now these gimmick glasses and contacts no longer are necessary, for a technologically perfect procedure has been developed to correct nearsightedness. It's called radial keratotomy, the RK we have waxed so enthusiastically.

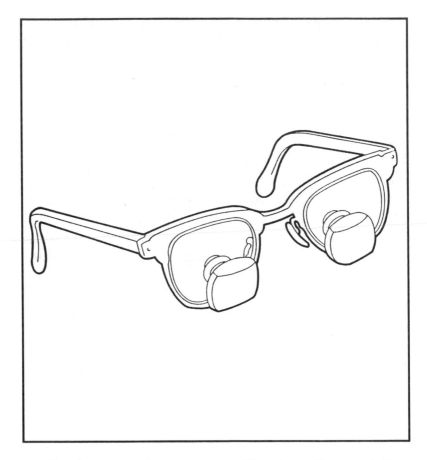

Eyeglasses perform a variety of functions from assisting people to see better, to protecting your eyes from the sun to enhance one's appearance. Pictured above is a special pair of magnifying binocular glasses. They are used in occupations which require close work, such as dentistry, surgery, or even on assembly lines where workers handle minute objects.

Chapter 4

The Permanent Correction of Nearsightedness

Appearing about twenty years younger than her present age of 46, Melony Carson of New York City does everything possible to remain youthful and beautiful. She is tall and willowy, uses cosmetics like an artist, and has long, blond hair.

Melony can't wear contact lenses comfortably because of an acute sensitivity reaction to them, and she disdains using eyeglasses because she believes they make her seem old and ugly. But corrective lenses or other vision aids are a necessity for the woman inasmuch as she is exceedingly nearsighted. If Melony tries to go without help from viusal aids, she just can't make out the details of anything in her surroudings. Her vision in each eye is only 20/400 or less. Despite her not wanting to, spectacles or some other corrective aids are devices she must wear at her job as a legal secretary and receptionist.

Greeting clients and other visitors for her attorney employer has the woman repeatedly removing her eyeglasses. She does this for two reasons: for sight and for vanity. Wearing a correction for myopia is an obstacle to her recognizing anything at close range. The woman can't make out the features of office visitor's faces so that she must take off the spectacles. In turn, Melony would never allow someone to check out her looks while she is wearing eyeglasses, especially if that someone is a handsome man, so off come the visual aids as soon as the outside door opens. Of course, she hated even the idea of resorting to bifocals.

In June 1984, Ms. Carson brought her eye problems to her ophthalmologist. Her doctor suggested that the eye surgery known as radial keratotomy (RK), today's fastest growing advance in eye care since contact lenses, be carried out. It was the ophthalmologist's concept, tailored to this woman's visual, psychological, occupational, and social needs, that he perform the surgery on only one of her eyes. In this way, she could have distance vision with lens correction from the operated eye, and still use the unoperated for near work, again without correction.

Of course, the eye surgeon explained, "It will take considerable practice to coordinate your eyes in order to be able to use them alternately, as you desire." Melony Carson was strongly motivated to give the procedure a try. Radial keratotomy for the left eye was scheduled the next week, and Melony's eye coordination practice continued for a month, thereafter.

The concept worked quite well. RK for one eye has totally satisfied both her viusal and vanity needs. As far as vision is concerned, Melony Carson will remain 26 years old forever.

Unlike Melony who merely looks 26, Samuel Muldoon, also of New York City, really is 26 years old. He earns a fine living as a junior business executive and certified public accountant with one of the major oil companies. Sam enthusiastically plays squash and tennis almost daily, and his game is so good that the young man is in demand with older executives as a workout partner.

His skill with a racket has been instrumental in getting Sam into some of the best sports clubs in the city. Unfortunately, the junior executive must wear eyeglasses when he plays racket sports because he is about minus four (-4.00) diopters myopic. Spectacles do get in his way, he feels, and contact lenses invariably pop out and are lost during the course of the various racket games.

In July 1984, Sam Muldoon wondered out loud to his ophthalmologist about what might be done to correct his nearsightedness so that lenses no longer would be required.

Exhaustive studies were made by the eye surgeon for carrying out an exact radial keratotomy. Unabashedly, Muldoon expressed how impressed he was by the careful measurements and other tests the operation demands of any ophthalmologist executing RK.

The next day, in just twelve minutes of actual operating time, the doctor completed the first RK without any pain or bleeding from Muldoon's right eye. Three weeks later the left eye was corrected. In two months more, the junior executive was back playing tennis and squash without the need for any corrective lenses. No longer is he nearsighted, and Samuel Muldoon reports that he's hitting the ball better than ever.

Robert McQueen of Danbury, Connecticut, 32, works in one the highly technical industries situated in that suburban city. He is the victim of moderately severe myopia with -5.00 diopters in each eye. For McQueen, contact lenses and eyeglasses are uncomfortable to wear. He's tried all kinds of corrective lenses and spent a lot of money doing it.

One day in May, 1984, while visiting his eye doctor, McQueen noticed the doctor owned a piece of sophisticated high tech equipment. It was a computer, invented by Philadelphia ophthalmologist Frederic B. Kremer, M.D., which delivers a surgical plan for radial keratotomy using multiple regression analysis. The computer interested the patient and he asked lots of questions about RK.

The doctor explained that "each eye and each patient presents a different series of problems. Cookbook surgery cannot be used with this RK technique." Then the eye surgeon showed McQueen the corneal thickness measuring device, the pachymeter, which meters the exact size of the cornea using sound waves. "Could you do the RK procedure to correct my nearsightedness?" Bob McQueen asked.

The following week he returned for a preoperative workup to determine if he was a candidate for RK. Intraocular pressures were taken. Corneal curvature was measured. Refraction was measured. Endothelial cell counts were done. All other necessary preoperative tests were carried out. Bob definitely was a RK candidate.

Without any requirement for the patient to spend $700 for use of a hospital surgical room, the surgeon carried out the procedure in his exurban office the next week. The right eye was operated on first, and three weeks later the left eye was also corrected. The man's vision is now 20/20 in the right eye and 20/25 in the left. He is nearsighted no

79

more and doesn't have to wear eyeglasses or contacts ever again.

Twenty-eight-year-old Janet Icons of Long Island, New York, is engaged to a man who had undergone RK for both eyes about four years ago. There was a time when his myopia was severe, but a Baltimore eye surgeon operated on him and obtained excellent results. He no longer wears any corrective lenses.

Ms. Icons' fiancee virtually insisted that the young woman experience RK surgery also. He believed that it was silly to remain myopic because the condition can be made right in such a simple matter. Consequently, she visited the eye surgeon early in July 1984 to have the operation performed.

The ophthalmologist, seeing that Janet was only moderately nearsighted, warned her that she should not undergo radial keratotomies just to please her boyfirend. She decided to have the preoperative measurements completed anyway, and was amazed at the number of tests carried forward prior to accomplishing the correction. The Kremer computer read-out told the eye surgeon just what should be the depth of the cornea cuts for the patient. Janet requested the doctor to do the permanent surgical technique for her myopia if she was a candidate. She was, and he did.

In a few days, the RK achieved an excellent correction of Janet Icons' left eye. "The procedure is so simple and without discomfort," she remarked immediately afterward. There was pleasure and surprise in her voice. Six weeks later when the right eye was fixed, as well, her vision had been improved to 20/20 in each of the operated eyes. Janet declared, "My fiancee was absolutely right in recommending radial keratotomy. He really loves me."

What is the Eye Problem Called Myopia?

It is estimated by the United States National Eye Institute that every fourth adult around the world is affected to some degree by myopia, the medical name for nearsightedness. Myopia is a condition in which parallel rays of light are focused in front of the retina, the consequence of an error in refraction of or elongation of the globe of the eye, causing nearsightedness.

To explain more fully: In normal vision, light rays entering the eye are bent by the cornea, bent and inverted by the lens, and come to focus on the retina, the sensitive membrane at the back of the eye that receives images and transmits them through the optic nerve to the brain, where the image is turned right side up. In nearsighted eyes, images fall short, coming to focus in front of the retina.

Myopia is expressed medically in terms of diopters. If a patient has one diopter (-1.00 D) of nearsightedness, this means the farthest focus of the eyes is one meter (about three feet) from his or her eyes. If the patient has two diopters (-2.00 D) of nearsightedness, his or her farthest point of vision is half a meter from the eyes; with three diopters (-3.00 D) of such myopia, the far point is a third of a meter; with four diopters (-4.00D), the far point is one-fourth of a meter. In other words, the person having nearsightedness of -4.00D or one-fourth of a meter as his or her far vision can see clearly only to a distance of approximately nine inches. Between -1.00 D and -4.00 D is in the average or "usual" range of myopia.

Myopia consists essentially of two types; (1) usual myopia, in which the eyeball is longer than normal and with a cornea that is too refractive for which the patient may be wearing concave lenses in order to see at a distance, (2) the pathologic higher degree of myopia in which the patient may have approximately -7.00 diopters of "high myopia." Then unusual changes begin to become apparent to the examining ophthalmologist, due to excessive stretching and elongation of the eyeball.

Using an instrument called the ophthalmoscope,

the eye doctor sees the interior of your eye by using a beam of light directed inside. He observes along the spot where the beam falls and checks for a white crescent (conus) around the optic nerve. When stretching of the eyeball from high myopia becomes too great for the retina and choroid to withstand, the choroid becomes thinned and a large, whitish, yellow area of tissue degeneration is seen. The stretching produces cracks and even areas of wasting in the macula. At times a small red or black spot resulting from hemorrhage in the fovea may be observed. This is bad because it abolishes central vision and is referred to as a "Fuch's dot." Thus, while nearsightedness is a mechanical condition of the eyes, it can bring on an abnormal physiological change resulting in disease.

How Does Radial Keratotomy Help?

The operation known as radial keratotomy is performed by microsurgery to correct usual myopia and sometimes high myopia. Its technique is precise and the result is unique.

Corrective lenses work for nearsightedness by changing the angle of the entering light rays so that they come to a focus on the retina. RK seeks the same end, but by a different mechanism: by changing the curvature of the cornea.

The curvature change is carried out under local anesthesia, merely using a liquid anesthetic dropped on the eye. The patient remains alert or he or she may choose to be sedated with a tranquilizer. Only one eye is operated on at a time; the other may be done two to three weeks later. The eye is kept open during surgery with a delicate clamp. There is no pain, no bleeding, and the slowest surgeon could take as long as twenty minutes to compete the entire operation. An RK finished in ten or twelve minutes is standard.

The operator marks the cornea with a special instrument to outline the visual center, which is left untouched, and a tiny sort of cookie-cutter tool with eight spokes radiating like the spokes of a wheel is pressed into the cornea to produce indentations the surgeon can follow to make his incisions.

Working with the aid of a microscope and using a tiny diamond blade with a guard to gauge the depth of incision, the doctor makes tiny cuts from the center outward. The length of such micro-incisions vary from case to case and don't fully penetrate the cornea, only about three-fourths of its thickness, depending on the degree of the patient's myopia. By cutting from seventy percent to ninety percent into the cornea's half-millimeter depth, the corneal tissue becomes weakened. In-

RADIAL KERATOTOMY

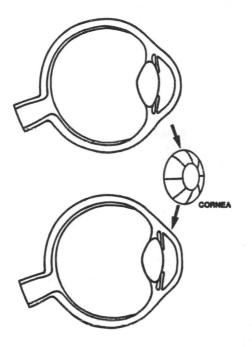

In myopia, as shown in the uppermost drawing, the cornea bulges outward abnormally causing the image to form in front of the retina instead of exactly on it. Consequently, the ophthalmologist performing radial keratotomy makes eight cuts, more or less, as shown in the middle drawing, into but not through the cornea leaving a clear central zone untouched. Thus, as indicated in the drawing below by the square surface of the outer portion of the eye, the cornea tends to flatten somewhat, in accordance with the premeasured requirement of your vision correction as determined by the eye surgeon.

ternal eye pressure then causes the edge of the cornea to bulge slightly, which flattens the central area. Thus, the visual center drops after surgery, resulting in improved vision.

After the operation, antibiotic drops are used and the eye is patched, to remain so for twenty-four hours. Healing of the epithelium takes place within this time. The sensation of an irritated eye may persist for two weeks or so, but reportedly is not particularly troublesome. Most RK patients return to work a day or two after the operation.

With the change in curvature, the corrected cornea bends the light rays at a new angle. The result is improved vision because images are now focused farther back, on the retina. The operation may take place in the ophthalmologist's office; hospitalization is not required. The degree of permenent correction achieved is usually evident by the third postoperative month. Follow-up examinations are carried out to monitor the patient's corneal measurements and to note how the eye is responding.

The Effectiveness of RK

Referring to statistics based on studies of 15,126 patients who underwent RK in the United States, Robert H. Marmer, M.D., in private practice of ophthalmology in Atlanta, in June 1984, told Ophthalmology Times, the monthly magazine distributed to the entire ophthalmic profession, "Radial keratotomy appears to be safe and effective, judging from results with patients followed up for five years in the United States and more than ten years in the Soviet Union."

Dr. Marmer further stated, "Eighty-five percent of patients with -2.00 diopters (D) to -6.00 D of myopia, and even some with up to -8.00 D, have achieved a visual acuity of 20/40 or better. Above the predictive area of -10.00 D (definite high myopia) this figure does not hold true. Such patients should be advised that they may not be corrected completely by surgery. A -10.00 D patient might expect reduction to -3.00 D of myopia, although complete emmetropia (parallel rays of light, when the eye is at rest, are focused exactly on the retina) is possible. Hopefully, the majority of patients will not require optical correction postoperatively."

Radial keratotomy is appropriate for a wide range of patients since it can be tailored to meet individual needs. "This procedure works because the cornea heals in a new position. There is always an initial overcorrection to allow for postoperative regression. The degree of correction and compensation can be varied as needed by applying a formula to data on each patient. Special keratotomy patterns are sometimes used when a patient has a significant amount of astigmatism, "said Dr. Marmer.

He noted that RK may not always provide adequate correction for patients whose major daily activities involve work requiring near vision such as draftsmen or artists, or for those people over forty years of age. "Because older patients tend to be presbyopic, they will probably continue to require spectacle correction for near vision," said the ophthalmologist. "Those patients in this age range who understand and accept this are defintely candidates for radial keratotomy surgery. This is dramatically illustrated by the 47-year-old ophthalmologist on whom I performed bilateral radial keratotomy surgery and who now functions wihtout optical correction in his busy surgical practice."

In September 1983, Spencer P. Thornton, M.D., director of research for the Eye Foundation of Tennessee located in Nashville, reported that a high success rate had been obtained in a series of patients undergoing radial keratotomy for myopia. "An overall average of 73 percent of our patients having between 2 diopters and 18.5 D of myopia attained 20/40 or better uncorrected vision," he stated to the Biennial Canadian Contact and Intraocular Lens Conference in Toronto. Jean Robertson, a registered nurse and certified ophthalmic technician, assisted him in the collection data.

The series consisted of two hundred consecutive patients who underwent operations after November 1979. The lowest degree of myopia was -2.00 D, while the highest amount was -18.5 D. The longest follow-up period was 3.5 years. All patients in the series were followed for at least one year. Approximately 71 percent of the patients had preoperative uncorrected vision of 20/400 or worse.

"Among those patients who had less than 6D of myopia preoperatively, approximately 80 percent had improvements in vision to 20/40 or better without correction," Dr. Thornton said. Postoperative acuity of 20/15 to 20/25 was achieved in 43 percent of the patients, and 75 percent of the total patient population was within +1.00 D or -1.00 D of emmetropia.

In patients with myopia of -3.00 D or less, 86 percent had postoperative vision of 20/40 or better. Seventy-six percent of patients whose myopia ranged from -3.00 D to 05.00 D attained 20/40 vision or better postoperatively. In those with -5.00 D to -8.00 D of myopia, 68 percent attained 20/40 or better. Half of those patients with nearsightedness above -8.00 D attained 20/40 vision or better.

Only 2 percent of all patients had overcorrections of myopia that were more than +2.00 D of hyperopia (farsightedness) after one year. "There were no surgery-related complications that resulted in a loss of best-corrected visual acuity of more than one line in any case," Dr. Thornton said. He noted that some patients have lost enough improvement in visual acuity to warrant a second operation. However, no patient has lost all improvement. Second operations were performed either to add more incisions or to deepen existing ones, he added.

Why RK Becomes Necessary in Some Situations

Some critics of the radial keratotomy procedure maintain that it is cosmetic surgery, thus relegating it to a lesser role as a method of treatment for the eye. Dr. Michael R. Deitz of Kansas City argues that the benefits RK are first, functional improvement and second (though less important), cosmetic improvement. "Function appears to be far more important to the patients I have treated," he told the August 1980 Kerato-Refractive Society Symposium on RK. "They're far more interested in how well they see the world then how well the world sees them."

Dr. Deitz stressed the importance of unaided good vision in times of emergency. Automobile drivers with high myopia cannot afford to lose their corrective glasses while driving in high-risk situations. Or, in the event of fire while asleep at a hotel, a guest who was nearsighted might be hard pressed to make his way to the exit, Dr. Dietz pointed out.

A Necessary and Beneficial RK

Nickolas Totora of Springfield, Massachusetts lay on the operating table at the Massachusetts General Hospital, the sixty-seventh Boston metropolitan area person to undergo RK through the first quarter of 1984. Within fifteen minutes of the beginning of surgery, 20-year-old Nickolas was up and out of the operating room. He was anxious to "have a look at my new vision." His left eye had been cured of nearsightedness only a month before, and the right eye was the one done now.

"I had begun wearing eyeglasses at the age of two," the patient said, "and they didn't do more than act as a crutch. My vision was getting worse. After entering college, my lenses were so thick, I had to put them on before getting out of bed in the morning to see my way clearly to the bathroom. I couldn't read any of my textbooks without them. Once I was giving a speech to the student body and one of the lenses fell out of its frame. I had to abort the speech. Was I ever embarrassed. That's when I prevailed on my parents to pay for this double session of operations. I don't want to wear eye-glasses anymore."

As he spoke, Nickolas reached for a pair of eyeglass frames in which the left lens had been poked out. He had been using just the right lens for his eyes and seeing normally without the lens for his left. NIckolas pushed against the right lens and popped it out of its frame. "I won't be needing these at all anymore," the young man said.

Looking at the eye first operated on, through a slit lamp, we saw the right radial cuts that had been made in Nickolas' cornea. They were periph-eral to that part of it covering the iris, showing only as faint lines which were minute scars of healing.

After the operation, an antibiotic eyedrop is used and the patient is ordinarily patched for twenty-four hours, as mentioned earlier. But this patient declined so much as a bandage for the newly operated eye. The bandage was not put on so as to permit Nickolas the self-testing of his vision after surgery.

His first comment as he covered his corrected left eye and looked at a wall chart out of his newly cured right was, "Oh boy, I can read even the small letters on line 8, D E F. . ."

The rate of success averages 85 percent among all of the eye surgeons performing radial keratotomy. Some are getting as high as 92 percent successes with their formerly myopic patients, but others report a 55 percent success ratio. As with other medical procedures, the result of the operation depends on the skill of the surgeon, his technique, and the severity of the patient's nearsightedness. Some doctors are taking only more difficult cases so that their success rates are lower. Others accept just the easier myopics so as to have better success rates.

In the postoperative management period, a slit lamp followup examination is essential. Corneal curvatures must be measured periodically, and temporary glasses are sometimes used during the recovery period. Additionally, for those patients who don't get a full correction of their myopia (for example a minus six diopter reduced to a minus two diopter), corrective lenses either as spectacles or contacts may still be required.

Some patients complain of the side effect of glare while driving at night, but this generally resolves by the end of two or three months. If a mild infection occurs, it is readily managed with medicated eye drops. Complete healing may take up to two months, during which the surgeon follows the patient's progress closely to assure the proper amount of corneal flattening. Sometimes the operation, is repeated to insure a perfect result. Other brief complications are redness and temporary sensitivity to light.

In the chapters to follow, we will give in-depth descriptions of the history, techniques, instrumentations, possible side effects, complications, contraindications, visual benefits, and everything else you will wish to know about radial keratotomy.

Chapter 5

The Evolution of Radial Keratotomy

An obstetrician-gynecologist practicing in Nashville, Tennessee, Jill F. Chambers, M.D., had both high myopia and astigmatism before undergoing radial keratotomy, but following the operation she reports vision improvement to 20/15.

"My vision was 20/200 preoperatively, "said Dr. Chambers. "My glasses were a problem when I was performing microscopic surgery or using a larparoscope. (A laparoscope is a surgical instrument comprising an illuminated viewing tube that is inserted through the abdominal wall to enable the surgeon to view the organs in the abdomen.) The obsterician-gynecologist recalled that she could not tolerate hard or soft contact lenses, and skin lesions were forming under the rims of her heavy glasses.

"It was a big decision to let someone operate on

my eyes for an investigational operation," Dr. Chambers admitted. "I really had it with corrective lenses, though, I felt that I had tried every kind of contact lens made. One thing that appealed to me was learning that the operation came about from the observation that trauma to the eye that flattened the cornea could reduce nearsightedness."

Dr. Chambers first read of surgical correction for myopia and astigmatism in newspapers and then asked for more information from Spencer P. Thornton, M.D., her Nashville ophthalmologist. "Dr. Thornton gave me information on the operation," she said, "and also allowed me to watch him perform the surgery."

Eight-incision radial keratotomy was done on her left eye in August 1982, and on her right eye in October 1982. "I was pregnant at the time, so I did not allow Dr. Thornton to use any sedation, just local anesthesia," she noted. During the eight weeks between the procedures, she unsuccessfully tried wearing glasses with a plano (flat and uncorrected) lens over the operated eye.

"I had my surgery on a Friday; I went back to work on Monday; and I was performing surgery the following Wednesday," said Dr. Chambers. During this period, she did have some eyestrain and headaches, "but not enough to keep me from working." However, with only one corrected eye, she found she could not read. These difficulties were eliminated when the second eye was operated on. Glare and photosensitivity were minor problems while the incisions healed, she pointed out, but these resolved within a few weeks after surgery. "My vision is now 20/15 in both eyes, with no astigmatism."

Postoperative results have been especially gratifying for Dr. Chambers, in part because her astigmatism has been completely corrected. "I see details now that I had never seen with contact lenses or eyeglasses. I had never seen each leaf on a tree before, for instance," she said. Surgery has also become easier for her to accomplish for her patients. "I am able to perform more detailed surgical techniques because my astigmatism is corrected. I would recommend the precedure almost without reservation."

In fact, she did recommend RK to a colleague and he had it done. Dr. Spencer Thornton also performed radial keratotomies for the second phycician, John Witherspoon, M.D., an otolaryngologist in private practice, also in Nashville, Tennessee. Vision for Dr. Witherspoon was about 20/400 before RK, and he mentioned that he had worn eyeglasses since early childhood.

Originally, this ear and throat specilist heard about RK at an outpatient surgery clinic where he performed surgery in his specialty. He then talked to Dr. Chambers, who told him of her successful experiences with undergoing the eye correction. Dr. Thornton performed eight-incision RK on Dr. Witherspoon's left eye in March 1983, and on the right eye in May 1983. "My vision is about 20/20 in the left eye," he reported. "My right eye was recently tested, and the vision is now fairly close to that in the other eye." No problems with excessive glare or fluctuation were evident, he said.

Both Drs. Chambers and Witherspoon, as knowledgeable patient-physicians, have recommended the procedure to friends and other physicians.

RK's Accidental Discovery

The modern techniques for radial keratotomy evolved about twelve years ago out of a Moscow schoolyard fight, when a punch shattered 16-year-old Boris Petrov's spectacles. Proponents of RK, who call that punch "a blow heard round the ophthalmological world," say it may have given 60 million nearsighted Americans and almost a billion Europeans, Africans, Asians, North Americans, South Americans, Australians, and New Zealanders the chance to throw away their eyeglasses and contact lenses forever.

How did this important medical breakthrough

arise from a schoolyard scrap? "Young Petrov suffered from nearsightedness," explained Svyatoslav N. Fyodorov, M.D., who was then professor of ophthalmology and director of the Moscow Scientific Research Laboratory of Experimental Eye Surgery, but has since been elevated to medical director of the entire Microsurgical Eye Institute of Moscow. "When he was punched, glass fragments slashed his cornea. It was cut superficially-it would heal. But three days later, he told me, 'Doctor, I have beautiful vision!' The glass shards, it appeared, had 'operated' on his eye. I thought, well, if a boy can treat myopia with his fist, maybe we can treat it surgically." Thus, Dr. Fyodorov developed the RK procedure and eventually introduced it worldwide.

In 1972, using a computer and refined microsurgery, the Russian discovered that he could alter the optical power of a rabbit's eyes with sixteen incisions radiating like the spokes of a wheel away from the cornea's delicate central optical zone. By 1974, Dr. Fyodorov was ready for the first test on humans. So was 24-year-old Misha, a very nearsighted limousine driver at the clinic. Misha's two operations were complete successes. With his colleagues at the Moscow laboratory, Dr. Fyodorov has since performed radial keratotomies on some 7,000 Russian patients with excellent and almost predictable results.

Prior to Fyodorov's discovery, however, Professor T. Sata, M.D. of Tokyo, Japan, an ophthalmologist (now deceased), published two papers. One was printed in the 1952 Japanese medical journal Rinsho. Ganka, volume 6, pages 209-211, under the title "Experimental Study of Anterior and Posterior Half-Corneal Incisions for Myopia." Then again, following his performance of the operation on human patients, in volume 36, on page 823 of a 1953 issue of the *American Journal of Ophthalmology*, Dr. Sato described and also illustrated a method of reshaping the corneal surface to effect flattening of the curvature. He wrote, "This new surgical approach to myopia (anterior and posterior half-corneal incisions) is a proven, safe method which definitely cures or adequately alleviates over 95 percent of all cases of myopia in Japan."

Dr. Sato's idea was to produce a weakening of the outside of the cornea so as to cause a steepening of the peripheral curve and a compensatory flattening of the central curavature. His method called for both external and internal partial thickness incisions with a standard six millimeter optic zone. Despite his glowing report, the procedure fell into disrepute because results were poor. Moreover, the technique was difficult to perform. Corneas became cloudy. This was not good for the patient's vision. The method was abandoned.

Such an inauspicious beginning has generated

considerable opposition from more conservative American ophthalmologists to the adoption of the highly advanced Fyodorov technique which is utilized today. Writing in Refractive Corneal Surgery: The Correction of Aphakia, Hyperopia and Myopia, which comprises the Fall, 1983 edition of International Ophthalmology Clinics, volume 23, number 3, pages 93-118, Leo D. Bores, M.D. of Santa Fe, New Mexico, one of Dr. Fyodorov's disciples, points out: "Our better understanding of the role of the endothelium in maintaining corneal clarity coupled with advances such as the operating microscope, ultrasonic pachymeter, and more precise methods of measuring corneal curvature has changed not only the performance of the procedure but also its potential."

Dr. Bores' chapter in this journal under the title, "Historical Review and Clinical Results of Radial Keratotomy," goes on to say: "Fyodorov recognized the shortcomings of Sato's technique and his imitators and made several important changes in the corneal refractive procedure. These changes were: (1) varying the size of the optical zone from 2.0 to 6.0 mm; (2) making all incisions from the external surface of the cornea; (3) using a surgical microscope during the procedure; (4) basing incision depth on actual measurements of corneal thickness (using optical pachymetry) and checking the depth of the incisions with specially constructed

101

gauges or dipsticks; and (5) using ultrasharp disposable razor fragments to make the incisions." Thus, the modern techniques of refractive surgery for the cornea had been launched.

In all fairness to ophthalmological pioneers, it must be mentioned that even before Dr. Sato's failed effort, other physicians had attempted to alter the distance light rays must travel to project on the retina of elongated eyeballs. Publishing in the 1869 issue of Albrechtvon Graefes Arch. Klin. Exp. Ophthalmol., Dutch ophthalmologist Dr. H. Snellen discussed the possibilities of correcting corneal astigmatism. In 1948, Dr. W.H. Bates suggested an operation to correct astigmatism in an article published in the Archives of Ophthalmology. He reported on operatory modifications and furnished a number of cases. Four years later, Dr. L. Lans did the same, also publishing in the Albrecht von Graefes Arch. Klin. Exp. Ophthalmol.

Finally, sandwiching his published report between Drs. Sato and Fyodorov, Jose I. Barraquer, M.D. of Bogota, Columbia, almost thirty years ago developed the two classic procedures, keratophakia and keratomileusis. These were the primary techniques in refractive surgery until radial keratotomy came along. Dr. Barraquer's report on the subject appeared in 1964 in the Archives of the Soceity of American Ophthalmology. Herbert E. Kaufman, M.D., Director of Louisana State University Eye Center, and Marguerite B. McDonald, Assistant Professor of Ophthalmology, Louisana State University Eye Center, described the two Barraquer operations in the June 1, 1984, issue of Ophthalmology Times. Drs. Kaufman and McDonald wrote: "Keratophakia involves splitting the cornea in half with a microkeratome instrument and putting a small lathed button of donor cornea between the halves. The top of the original cornea is then sewn back into position. This technique was used on extremely hyperopic (farsighted) patients or on aphakes (people lacking crystalline lenses) who were unable to use spectacles or contact lenses.

"In keratomileusis, the cornea is spilt, and the top layer is removed and shaped on a cryolathe (a tiny grinder that simultaneously freezes tissue). The reshaped tissue is then reattached without the addition of any donor material . . The main disadvantage of these techniques was that they could be performed by only a few surgeons. . . use of the microkeratome requires an extraordinary amount of skill and practice, and the cryolathe is an expensive device. In addition, practitioners had to travel to Bogota in the early years to learn the techniques directly from Dr. Barraquer. . . This situation led to the development of more accessible techniques. . ."

Refractive Eye Surgery Comes to the United States

The new surgical procedure for curing near-sightedness involving tiny multiple incisions on the cornea which was developed by Soviet Dr. S.N. Fyodorov did not win acceptance in the United States with the speed of vodka. Early in 1976, Dr. Leo D. Bores visited Dr. Fyodorov to study the surgeon's lens implant technique and was amazed at the results he was getting for the correction of myopia.

Dr. Bores describes what he witnessed this way: "My initial reaction was one of disbelief. A reaction that I'm sure everyone experiences when first exposed to this procedure. After all, it seemed rather a bizarre solution to the eyeglass problem." In addition, I was familiar with Sato's work. It hadn't worked for Sato, why should it work for Fyodorov? Could this be another Russian reinvention?

But Drs. Bores and Fyodorov became fast friends. They spoke together "heart-to-heart" (In Russian that's "dusha-dusha"). "Therefore, when he explained this procedure to me," Dr. Bores continued, "I was disposed to believe him, despite my misgivings. I was allowed to examine the patients without interference. They all had vision ranging from 20/15 to 20/30 unaided (after undergoing

104

RK). My examination of records showed that pre-operatively they all had 20/100 vision or less unaided. And if the records were correct, there was no question that their corneas had become flatter as a consequence of the surgery."

Dr. Bores then examined the next group of patients before they underwent RK. He observed the surgeries. His examination of them post-operatively indicated undoubtedly that their corneas had become flatter. Next, Dr. Fyodorov suggested that Dr. Bores try his hand at accomplishing the correction for patients. The following day they did six cases together. One eye of each patient was corrected. A week later the other eye was done for the same six people.

"In each case, flattening occurred and the myopia vanished," said Dr. Bores. "Furthermore, the patients that I had examined the previous week had returned and were examined again. They were still flat. Needless to say, I was impressed; I was also scared because if this operation really worked, it should be introduced into the United States. The potential of this procedure was enormous."

Because of fear of colleague criticism of RK saying it was too risky, too variable, too unpredictable, and wouldn't last, Dr. Bores held off its performance in this country. Dr. Fyodorov visited Detroit, in the fall of 1976 to give a lecture at the

Kresge Eye Institute on the topic of RK. The physician response was polite but indifferent.

Dr. Bores later returned to Moscow with a retinue of other American eye surgeons, in May 1977. He again examined the patients upon which he had operated the year before. They were still seeing well without viusal aids. He also examined the records of some othe earlier cases performed at the Moscow Scientific Research Laboratory of Experimental Eye Surgery. There were no regressions, no infections, no dystrophic changes. "Now," said Fyodorov, "You will do?"

Bores didn't "do" because of continuing anxiety about peer review. The influences of American medical schools and the hosptial residency system of medical teaching tends to remove physician's personal creativity. It represses the physician's inclination to accept any innovation without great resistance. Most doctors usually follow the state medical society's party line which scoffs at something new unless it undergoes "double-blind testing" or randomized studies. Innovation gets discouraged.

But when Fyodorov showed Bores, in the spring of 1978, records of the patients upon which the American had performed surgery two years before, the Russian couldn't be denied. Bores' Russian patients' excellent and sustained results coupled with the proof of good effects of four years of follow-ups on almost two hundred others, did it. "I had to get off dead center," declared Leo Bores, M.D.

In November 1978, on a 34-year-old American woman, Dr. Bores performed the first radial keratotomy in the United States. Two weeks later he corrected the woman's other eye. In January 1979, he presented the patient at Grand Rounds of his hospital and showed a film of the technique that had been produced while he had been performing the surgery. Dr. Bores also laid before his colleagues all of the existing Russian data about RK. Their response? ZERO! The one question asked by his colleagues was, "Isn't this the Sato procedure?"

Deciding to do his own thing, Bores set aside his anxiety about colleague criticism and performed RK on any patients whom he believed would benefit from the procedure and who asked for it. He constructed a protocol for other ophthalmologists to follow and set up the framework for a national study. In a copyrighted course that he created, Bores taught the operation to other eye surgeons. For example, William D. Myers, M.D. of Southfield, Michigan, Assistant Clinical Professor of Ophthalmology, Michigan State University, East Lansing, learned from Bores and, in turn, taught RK to Ronald A. Schachar, M.D., Ph.D., Director of the Texoma Eye Instistue of Denison, Texas, and his brother Les Schachar, M.D., Director, Eye Clinic at

107

nearby Gainesville, Texas. The four have performed some 3000 radial keratotomies to correct nearsighted eyes.

RK Becomes a Skill for Other American Eye Surgeons

Word of success for patients with myopia who experienced RK spread to other American eye surgeons. They either became disciples of the disciple Bores or traveled overseas to learn directly from the master.

In Denison, Texas, the Keratorefractive Society was formed. Its credo says it is "an independent, not-for-profit organization, founded for the express purpose of disseminating and facilitating the exchange of information concerning refractive alterations of the cornea and their surgical corrections. It serves as a repository for clinical data obtained under protocol by its members for purposes of analysis and professional evaluation.

"The Society's educational objectives are to stimulate research and investigation in keratorefraction in order to establish a broad base to evaluate the clinical applicability of techniques in this area. Such scientific exchange needs to be undertaken to avoid errors and controversy which have accompanied other popularized surgical techniques in recent years.

"The Society firmly believes that no single sub-group of surgeons should be the exclusive evaluator of any single procedure. It defends the right of any well-trained and responsibile ophthalmologist to undertake clinical investigations under well defined protocols with due regard for his patient's informed consent and rights.

"Membership in the Society is open to all ophthalmologists and scientists who have an interest in this area. Address all correspondence to Keratorefractive Society; P.O. Box 145; Denison, Texas 75020."

Jerry Zelman, M.D. of Hialeah, Florida, Norman O. Stahl, M.D., of Long Island, New York, an attending ophthalmologist at the New York Creative Surgery Center, New York City, and Herbert L. Gould, M.D. of White Plains New York, who is associate clinical professor of ophthalmology at New York Medical College, went to take training with Dr. Svyatoslav N. Fyodorov in Moscow. In a presentation before optometrists attending the 1980 Optifair meeting at the Hilton Hotel in New York City, Dr. Gould described how it is to take such Russian training.

Dr. Gould said: "In general, Russian medicine is behind American medicine but as far as ophthalmology is concerned, an anomoly exists. Russian ophthalmology is ahead of eye surgery practiced in the United States. Fyodorov supervises 200 eye surgeons working a 400-bed hospital devoted to the treatment of eye conditions. Most instruments are made in West Germany and much of the equipment is American-made. The waiting room of the Moscow Eye Institute looks like the reception area of Bellevue Hospital in New York City.

"The surgeons don't use rubber gloves for operating, just surgical scrubbing causing them to have the reddest hands you've ever seen. They do wear booties on their feet to cut down on infection. Operating tables stand side by side in the same room so that two cases performed by two surgeons will be operated on simultaneously. Patients are awake and alert. Anesthesia is merely with the use of drops. The heart of the whole RK operation is the micrometric knife; a knife with a micrometer on its back that tells the surgeon precisely-within a few microns-the amount of corneal tissue being incised. It helps an opthalmologist perform a more controlled operation."

Dr. Gould described to the Optifair audience, consisting mostly of optometrists, how Misha, the Russian chauffeur who works for the Moscow Eye Institute, meets important guests at the airport. Misha, you may recall, is the first person on whom Dr. Fyodorov performed radial keratotomy. It is Misha's habit, upon learning that the guest is a visiting ophthalmologist, to reach into the limou-

110

sine glove compartment and reveal his old, unused eyeglasses. They have lenses that look like the bottom of cola bottles and are the ones he had disposed of after undergoing RK. Not being near-sighted any longer, Misha's eyeglasses were just objects of curiosity for him. Now Misha wears no lenses at all. He drives without visual aids.

"A huge basket piled high with spectacles sits in one corner of the institue. It represents the result of successful RK's for people," Dr. Gould addition-ally explained. Patients throw away their spec-tacles following the operation.

Other American eye surgeons have taken train-ing with Fyodorov. Then they return to this country and teach the technique to fellow professionals. Moreover, Fyodorov has traveled to the United States about half-a-dozen times and participated in training sessions for American ophthalmolo-gists. They have awarded him various honors for his advancements in vision care.

What is the Cost of Undergoing This Myopia Repair?

The importance of vision to all Americans is dramatically indicated by certain facts. In 1972, the United States economy lost an estimated $1.5 billion in earnings due to visual disorders and disabilities, according to the National Advisory Eye

Council. In 1983, it was $5.2 billion.

From 350,000 to 600,000 Americans are currently estimated to be legally blind.

Among the chronic diseases which restrict the ability of Americans to lead productive lives, visual impairment ranks third after heart disease and arthritis.

One of every twenty preschool-age children has a vision problem, says the National Society to Prevent Blindness.

The National Eye Institute advises that almost one million U.S. citizens are visually impaired by injuries, nearly 2-1/4 million elderly Americans suffer vision loss from cataracts, about 95 percent of people over age 65 require some type of visual help, and one out of two of this country's residents wear corrective lenses.

Of all these statistics, the most significant is that practically all of the reported eye problems are connected in some way with refractive errors in the eye. The most common is nearsightedness with distorted and blurred vision. This common eye problem is correctable with radial keratotomy.

But the operation is not cheap. The preparation for the surgery is so extensive for each individual that ophthalmologists are charging for their time and training varying prices of $1,200 to $2,000 per eye, with the most commonly quoted cost being $1,500 for one surgery. Plus, there is a usual charge made by the hospital for the operating room of from $400 to $800.

The doctor's fee includes not only the surgery but also a schedule of follow up visits. The surgeon's follow up schedule sometimes, but not always, involves up to 36 months of attention. Some surgeons even offer four years or more of postoperative visits.

At the end of three months, the operated patient may be requested by his surgeon to visit another ophthalmologist, and frequently he or she does agree to see the other doctor for an eye examination and refractive measurements. At least six months of postoperative care will likely be included in the surgical fee. Keep in mind, however, that charges change along with practice, procedures. Nothing mentioned here about fees and postoperative attention must be though of as being written in stone.

The postoperative schedule of visits that the doctor and the patient obligate themselves to may be rather elaborate. They could follow a surprising frequency of appointments such as two days, seven days, two weeks, one month, two months, three months (the outside consultation), six months, nine months, twelve months, fifteen months, eighteen months, twenty-four months, thirty months, and thirty-six months.

The cost in time away from one's occupation is minimal, if any. For instance, your operation may be carried out on a Friday after work with recuperation, if necessary, over the weekend; you then return to work on Monday as if nothing happened. Less than two days will have been used for the correction.

Chapter 6

Reasons For Vision Impairment

A 27-year-old single, handsome, video camerman from San Diego named Ross Climo learned about the operative procedure to eliminate the need of soft contact lenses. Mr. Climo had been wearing contacts for five years to accommodate a moderately severe nearsightedness.

The hot Southern California weather with the excessive perspiration that it caused tended to fog the cameraman's visual aids and thus interfere with his earning a living. Camera work which he frequently performed sweltering in the field caused Climo eye irritation from using the contacts. He was experiencing difficulty with protein buildup between the lens and his eyeball. Such protein accumulation usually is a source of eye soreness for a contact lens user. It's accompanied by symptoms of burning, stinging, and redness. He, therefore,

115

attempted to avoid using lenses at any opportunity.

But Climo did require myopia correction because his visual acuity without it was 20/200 in the right eye and 20/300 in the left. It was either wear eyeglasses, which may have detracted from the way he appeared to women friends; continue with his soft contacts, which he was finding intolerable; or undergo the radial keratotomy (RK) surgery, which the cameraman chose to do.

Climo sought the services of a Diplomate of the American Board of Ophthalmology, Wendell P. Wong, M.D. who operates out of The Eye Surgery Center of Torrance, California. Dr. Wong has always believed that the average hospitalization period for eye patients (between three to five days) is too long and, consequently, too expensive. At the Eye Surgery Center, Dr. Wong emphasizes the importance of outpatient surgery. "In most cases," he says, "patients can have an operation and return to the comfort of their own home the same day, lessening their fears and anxieties, as well as greatly reducing costs." And this is how the nearsightness of Ross Climo was treated.

Learning that Climo's lifestyle included a lot of sports, including skin diving and surfing, besides the complications involving his wearing of lenses on the job, and then observing the man's eye

116

protein buildup, the ophthalmologist agreed that RK was the best way to correct his patient's eye problem. After the doctor explained options, alternatives, risks, and complications to Climo, the cameraman still insisted on having RK.

Dr. Wong consequently elected to perform RK on Climo's left eye first, using just topical anesthesia in the form of drops. Eight tiny insisions were made for the young man on April 5, 1984.

The day following Climo's left eye surgery his correction was 20/25 and one week later it improved even further to 20/20, where the patient's vision has now steadied. Ross Climo intends to have his right eye corrected when it's convenient for him. In the meantime, he never again requires any contact lens for his left eye. Dr. Wong has his patient visit for checkups at regular intervals and reports that the patient's operative result for nearsightedness remains perfect.

Nearsightedness Compared to Other Eye Problems

Unlike other possible eye problems, nearsightedness does not make its appearance overnight like the symptoms of an infectious disease; it comes on gradually and may go unnoticed until the victim can't see print on a page.

At the United States Naval Academy at Annapolis, for example, the first-year plebes arrive with good acuity, since it is a definite necessity for admission. By graduation, it's not uncommon for a quarter of the cadet class to have become nearsighted. They seem to acquire their myopia during their four years of study. In one class, over 50 percent ended up myopic.

It seems that myopia is on the increase. Traditional medicine considers the source of nearsightedness to be a fault in the curvature of the cornea and rarely an inherited elongation of the eyeball, combined with eyestrain and other overuse of the eyes. Before age ten, about 5 percent of all college students appear to become somewhat nearsighted.

As mentioned previously, nearsightedness is a refractive problem of light entering the eyeball. It is a mechanical difficulty - an optical distortion - as is farsightedness, astigmatism, and the type of farsightedness more mature people experience which is known as presbyopia. Most other eye difficulties are not mechanical in nature. They are actual infections, inherited disorders, or degenerative diseases. For instance, glaucoma is a degenerative disease characterized by a higher than normal pressure inside the eye (intraocular pressure). Because of similarities in optical distortion, sometimes eye diseases are mistaken for refractive problems when they are not.

This chapter is devoted to educating you about reasons for different kinds of vision impairment not related to refractive correction. Knowing about such disabilities as macular degeneration, trachoma, conjunctivitis, diabetic retinopathy, retinitis pigmentosa, and others will help you differentiate them from the problems of refraction.

Macular Degneration

The retina is capable of two kinds of vision: central and peripheral. With central vision you distinguish detail at close range as in reading and sewing, and at a distance as with following road signs. Peripheral vision allows you perception of your surroundings including objects and movement not in the direct line of sight. Peripheral vision prevents collisions with others when walking or driving.

Central vision is performed by the macula, the tiny spot in the center of each retina. In macular degeneration it is this minute area which deteriorates, gradually blurring and eliminating central vision but leaving most of the peripheral vision intact. The deterioration is more common in the aged from hardening of the arteries. Thus, macular degeneration is partial or total loss of the sensitive

119

macula area in the retina providing sight and color vision resulting in a reduced ability to see.

Sometimes macular degeneration occurs prior to old age, from hereditary or other causes not yet understood by medical science. If the disease is limited to one eye, the patient may continue to function normally. When the condition occurs in both eyes, functioning is altered and a reorientation of goals and work must be undertaken.

Treatment of macular degneration is administered with new technology using a focused laser beam. The treatment is not uncomfortable to the patient and often doesn't even require hospitalization. Optical devices known as low-vision aids also are used for macular degeneration. These are various types of magnifying lenses which provide enlarged images for the victim of macular degeneration.

Zinc and Macular Degeneration

Preliminary studies with zinc show that this trace metal may help prevent macular degeneration.

Dr. David A. Newsome of the Louisiana State University Eye Center in New Orleans conducted a study among 151 patients. Eighty of these people took 100 mg zinc tablets twice a day. The others received a placebo—a harmless pill which would promote no effects on the eyes.

After two years, these who took zinc had significantly less vision loss and fewer adverse retinal changes than those who received the placebo.

A larger study involving up to 1,000 patients is planned for the near future and this should help determine if zinc is really good for the eyes.

Zinc is a relatively rare nutrient, and most people do not receive enough of it through their daily diet.

Test Yourself For Macular Degeneration

The grid on the opposite page with the tiny dot in the center is called the Amsler grid. By following the directions which follow, one may be able to detect macular degeneration, the disease which affects a person's central vision.

Place the Amsler grid on a bare wall or door in well-lighted room. The center dot should be at eye level.

Mark off a spot on the floor 14 inches from the chart and stand facing it. Your heels should be on the spot you have marked.

Wear your glasses only if they are prescribed for reading. Look at the dot with your left eye covered, then with your right eye covered. If the grid is blurred or contains any blank spots, consult your ophthalmologist.

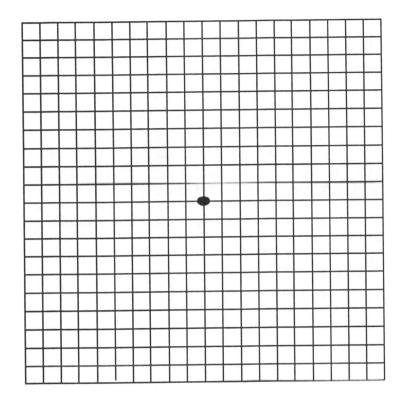

Trachoma

A chronic disease caused by an organism identified neither as a virus of a bacterium but with some properties of both, attacks the cornea and conjunctiva. The resultant disease is called trachoma. The World Health Organization states that trachoma "is the greatest single cause of progressive loss of sight" among third world nations. Over half a billion people suffer from the disease.

It spreads by close contact, especailly from one family member to the next. It may be carried by gnats and flies among those with poor hygiene, particularly in desert areas where lack of running water makes normal bathing impossible.

Trachoma treatment consists mainly of administering sulfonamide drugs, penicillin, and other antibiotic drugs. Following treatment and cure with antibiotics, upon the return of a formerly infected trachoma victim to similiar unhygienic conditions, he is likely to contract the disease again.

The trachoma germ gradually causes scarring of the conjunctiva which spreads to the cornea. Apart from the Indians of the Southwestern United States and among poverty-stricken Mexican-Americans, the disease is uncommon in this country. Its symptoms might be confused with glaucoma by someone unfamiliar with the two conditions.

Other Viral Infections

Herpes simplex is another disease that comes from microbial infection which may occur in the cornea. This herpes virus causes the common "cold sore" which may show up on the lips, for example.

Herpes zoster is a virus causing corneal problems as a result of its growth on the skin of the lids and in the nerves. This herpes infection can lead to drying of the cornea because of a decreased blind relfex.

Other forms of infection from bacterial invasion produce pus and scarring inside the eye called endophthalmitis. Very little room is present within the eye for this extra material, and the intraocular pressure can increase causing harmful effects to the nerves in the retina. The eye is a perfect culture medium for such invading organisms to grow. Trauma could be the cause of organism entry.

Conjunctivitis

The conjunctiva is a thin tissue that lies over the white part (sclera) of the eye. The medical term

125

which indicates inflammation that leaves the eye more red than white, called "pink eye" by many, actually is conjunctivitis. Other than cataracts and glaucoma, it is the most common of the acute and chronic eye diseases. About 750,000 cases of conjunctivitis are reported each year in the United States.

The signs and symptoms of conjunctivitis are distinct. Congestion and redness of the eye membrane, tearing and discharge of fluid during the night, and burning or stinging sensations are present. The eyelids may stay stuck together upon awakening in the morning as a result of the discharge.

Conjunctivitis comes from variable causes including infections, allergies, and physical agents such as too much sun, snow blindness, viewing electric welding arcs with the naked eye, and other physical irritants. Allergic conjunctivitis may develop from medications taken to offset hay fever. But most often it derives from bacterial or viral infection. In fact, the term "pink eye" is used in referring to a short-lasting but highly contagious conjunctivitis infection.

A person with conjunctivitis may feel mild, intermittent discomfort or more severe pain and sensitivity to light, depending on the seriousness of the infection or other cause. Decreased tear secretion may be the mildest of causes with a drying out of the conjunctiva producing slight irritation. If the drying continues for any length of time, less resistance to infection is available to the eye.

Conjunctivitis Treatments

Doctors often prescribe antibiotic drops for bacterial conjunctivitis. Frequently, antibiotics are also prescribed for viral infections to help prevent bacteria from invading, since bacteria may infect the conjunctiva weakened by the virus.

Instructions Chamomile
As a Wash: Steep 2 handfuls of the herb's flowers - either fresh or dried - in 4 quarts of boiling water for 10 minutes. Strain and allow to cool slightly before using. *Frequency of Use:* A few times throughout the day to help relieve conjunctivitis. *As a Compress:* Pour 2 cups boiling milk over a heaped tablespoon of the herb's flowers. Infuse briefly, strain and use warm. *Frequency of Use:* A few times throughout the day.

Consumers should be careful in the use of eye

drops which contain corticosteroids. While this hormonal-based remedy is effective, it can increase the pressure on the eye. Those with a herpes simplex eye infection, moreover, should not use the drops due to the very real possiblity of aggravating the infection.

A weak wash, made of the herb, Chamomile, relieves the inflamed eye and cures conjunctivitis, according to herbalists. Chamomile, one of the oldest and most versatile of medicinal herbs, was known to ancient Egyptian physicians, and is still widely used in Europe today. Chamomile can also be used in compress form to relieve "pink eye." See instructions on page 127.

Swedish Bitters, in addition to its curative powers over cataracts (as described on page 160), also relieves tired eyes. Apply the herbal mixture to the closed eyelid in the same manner as prescribed for the cataract treatment. See page 161 for the instructions making Swedish Bitters.

In many instances, removing the original irritant is sufficient treatment for conjunctivitis. For example, if sustained sunlight prompted the irritation, then keeping your eyes out of the sun for a while and wearing dark glasses are the best remedies.

Homeopathic Treatment

There are several homeopathic medicines which work well for conjunctivitis. Give a dose of the remedy three or four times daily for up to three days. Discontinue use when the symptoms show definite improvement.

Belladonna. This medicine can be given in the earliest stages of conjunctivitis, when the primary symptom is the sudden bright red, bloodshot inflammation of the membranes. The eyes may feel hot and they may throb, say homeopaths. Clear tears flow freely and light bothers the eyes.

Euphrasia (Eyebright). Use this remedy, homeopathic specialists say, in the presence of acrid, watery tears which burn the face. With time, the discharge may turn into a thick mucus, but it will not be opaque or yellow green. Euphrasia is a good choice when the eyes feel dry or when they feel as if there is sand or dust in them. Very often the eyes and the lids are red. This medication may also be used when there is an accompanying nasal drainage.

Apis. Homeopaths recommend use of this medicine when swelling of the conjunctivitis is extreme and heat aggravates the eyes. The conjunctival lining of the inner eyelid may be so swollen that it protrudes from behind the lid. The eyelids may be puffy as well as the areas above and below the lids. The eyes are red with gushing hot tears. This remedy is suggested also when the eyes burn or sting or when the discomfrot is worse in a warm room. Cold bathing of the eyes

---

Homeopathic Treatment (con't)

often relieves the irritation.

Pulsatilla. This is a recommended medicine for infections marked by the discharge of a thick yellow to greenish matter from the eyes, which does not irritate the skin. The eyes, however, may itch and burn, especially towards evening. The lid margins may also be extremely itchy. Pulsatilla is suggested when the symptoms are relieved by exposure to open air and by bathing the eyes in cold water.

Mercurius. This medicine is suggested by specialists when liquidy, irritating yellow to green discharge is present. It is usually less thick than that which calls for the use of Pulsatilla. Symptoms worsen at night, with the warmth of the bed as well as with the exposure of the glare of firelight. Mercurius is considered when whiteheads or scales around the eye or on the lids are present.

Hepar Sulph. Use this treatment if there is a thick puslike discharge or if discomfort increases with cold and decreases with exposure to warmth, specialists advise.

Signals of a More Serious Problem

Eyelid infections such as a stye, an infection of an eyelid oil gland can also occur. Eyelid infections are potenially serious since the organisms can

130

travel into blood vessels that connect directly with the brain. Antibiotic pills, lid scrubs, and hot compresses may be needed.

Sometimes conjunctivitis or an infection can lead to the discovery of another serious eye condition. For instance, Raphael Santina, 54, of Ocean City, New Jersey, who other than wearing reading glasses for his presbyopia, rarely had any eye problem, one day in July 1984 noticed some pain and redness in his left eye. Mr. Santini visited his family physician who prescribed an antibiotic drop as treatment. The doctor labeled the condition "conjunctivitis."

Sitting in the sun the next day, a Saturday, Santini continued to fell uncomfortable, although hardly as much as previously. Nevertheless, the man concluded that the eye drops were not very effective. Indeed, watching a movie on television that night had him experiencing rather sharp head pain above and around the left eye. And in the middle of the night deeper within the left eye it hurt even more. Early Sunday morning he called his family physician who recommended that he take aspirin, drink fluids, rest, and see an ophthalmologist at his first opportunity.

Monday morning the patient visited an ophthalmologist who found that Santini did have an infection but worse, he was the victim of acute narrow-angle glaucoma, a relatively rare form of the disease. The doctor prescribed various medications and drops which stabilized both infection and the glaucoma condition.

The eye surgeon explained that the entrances to drainage channels in Santini's eyes were narrower than normal. When he sat in a darker place such as in watching television, the man's pupils enlarged and closed the drainage channels to fluid leaving his eyes. When he went into the sun, the pupils constricted and the drainage channels were not as closed. Thus, the pressure inside his eyes was higher and the pain was more severe when he was in less light. Since the pressure was still too high, even in the bright sun, Santini experienced some pain, but not as much, when he went outside.

Raphael Santini underwent a surgical procedure to provide an alternate pathway for the fluid to leave his left eye. A month later he had the same procedure done on his other eye so that he wouldn't eventually experience the same problem with it. The man has not had any further difficulty. No permanent damage was done to the nerves. The conjunctivitis had actually saved his vision by forcing Santini to check the health of his vision by an eye doctor.

Diabetic Retinopathy

Portions of the eye are subject to illness with the retina being chief among them. Some conditions like *detached retina,* in which the retina comes loose from the choroid against which it normally rests, can be repaired if detached in time. Others, like the retinal damage - *diabetic retinopathy* - that is often seen in diabetes or in high blood pressure, may be extremely difficult to correct.

A major complication of diabetes, diabetic retinopathy is the fastest growing cause of blindness today. There are over ten million diabetics in the United States. Diabetes is the sixth most frequent cause of death among Americans. Of those who have been the victims of diabetes for eleven years or more, two-thirds will experience diabetic retinopathy. Moreover, it is present in more than 90 percent of those who have had diabetes for fifteen to twenty years. Diabetic retinopathy is reaching for equivalency with cataracts as the chief cause of blindness in this country.

"Retinopathy" simply means pathology or disease of the retina and roughly parallels the duration of diabetes. Diabetic retinopathy is a catchall term used to describe any of the various stages of retinal pathology caused by diabetes, including hemorrhages, thrombi, aneurysms, and scarring of the retinal tissue. Diabetes damages the circu-

133

lation by causing degeneration of the lining of walls of the blood vessels—first the microscopic capillaries, then the minute arteries and veins. Later, these little vessels become so weakened they occur most typically in the retina.

The retinal blood vessel changes and hemorrhages may result in new, abnormal blood vessels forming on the retina and growing into the clear, gel-like vitreous where they often hemorrhage. While this blood may eventually clear, the blood, blood clots, and blood vessels in the vitreous humor may cloud and affect sight. Massive retina detachment may also take place.

Treatment may consist of vitrectomy, in which the blood-filled vitreous is removed and replaced. Although an eye surgeon will be able to say whether the eye problem is the result of advanced or badly controlled diabetes, treatment must be aimed at the whole condition, not just at the retina.

The xenon arc laser is also proving extremely effective on this condition. It enables the surgeon to photocoagulate and destroy many of the disease-related abnormal blood vessels and aneurysms on an outpatient basis. This instrument is used primarily when a vitreous hemorrhage has already occurred. The laser's intense white light is focused on the retina after the pupil has been dilated.

The treatment, however, is not 100 percent effective. It cannot destroy the abnormal vessels which have formed above the retina or those directly on the optic nerve head.

The argon laser is also used in cases of diabetic retinopathy and can operate in only about a fifth of the space needed for an xenon beam as well as a fifth of the energy.

Warning Signals of Diabetic Retinopathy

Diabetics should be attuned to any changes in their eyesight, since diabetic retinopathy is, many times, a major complication of the disease. The following are some warning signs which might indicate development of the eye condition:

1) Sudden difficulty in reading. This may be a result of an excess of insulin in the system.

2) Rapid differences in the ability to see over the course of several days, a condition which is caused by high blood sugar levels.

3) Hazy or distorted areas in the field of view, which is the result of retinal tissue swelling or circulatory problems.

4) The sudden appearance of many spots. Often this is a signal of hemorrhage or detachment of the retina.

If you experience any of these symptoms, consult your ophthalmologist immediately.

Retinitis Pigmentosa

Authorities estimate that 100,000 Americans suffer from *retinitis pigmentosa,* a hereditary disease also of the retina. It usually is transmitted by the unaffected mother to her male child and often skips several generations. Over the victim's lifetime it gradually destroys the ability to see at night and reduces peripheral vision to leave only tunnel vision. This condition is due to changes in the retina.

The first symptoms appear in childhood or adolescence as night blindness and stumbling in the dark. The patient's range of vision is narrowed, so he cannot see to the sides or above or below the visual object. Eye surgeons examine the retina with an ophthalmoscope, an instrument used to look at the eye interior. They find areas of black-colored matter scattered throughout, but mostly to the sides. The small retinal arteries and veins are gradually obliterated and replaced by scars. The principal complications are physical injuries due to poor vision.

Vitamin A and Night Blindness

A clue to the cause of night blindness is *rhodopsin,* or visual purple, the pigment the eye uses for night vision.

One of the components of visual purple, *Vitamin A*, is not found in the other three pigments used to distinguish colors for daytime vision. A deficiency of Vitamin A, therefore, appears to inhibit the proper functioning of visual purple and prompts night blindness, without affecting one's vision during the day.

Recent studies seem to confirm Vitamin A's legendary reputation as the "eye vitamin." The symptoms of night blindness are greatly alleviated when treated with large doses of Vitamin A and the vegetable most commonly associated with it, the carrot. Carrots are the single most important natural source of beta-carotene, which the body uses to manufacture Vitamin A.

Deep orange fruits and vegetables such as broccoli, squash, apricots and peaches, also provide the body with beta-carotene, and are most beneficial when eaten fresh.

Many case histories are on record of people, plagued by night blindness, reporting dramatic improvements in their condition after adding carrots and beta-carotene to their diets. One of the easiest ways of getting more Vitamin A is by drinking carrot juice.

A typical example of the power of carrot juice is illustrated by the experience of a young mother suffering from night blindness. She avoided driv-

137

ing at night until her son's sudden illness. With her husband out of town on business, she was forced to drive her child to the hospital in the middle of the night. While she reached the hospital safely, and received the proper treatment for her son, the slow speed of her travel—an average of 15 miles per hour—disturbed her.

She vowed that she would never allow herself to be put in that position again. She began a regimen of drinking a quart of *Carrot Juice* a day, as well as feeding it to her family every morning. Her night vision improved in less than a month.

Instructions
Carrot Juice

Several raw carrots, cleaned well, but unpeeled. Place them in the juicer.

Frequency of Use: Drink liberally throughout the day.

Note: Carrot Juice's natural powers weaken with age, so it is best to drink the juice immediately after it is made.

Vitamin supplements are a useful way of boosting one's intake of Vitamin A.

It is a rare, special blend of powerful natural ingredients, proven successful in guarding against night blindness, eye fatigue, impaired vision and sensitivity to television, reading, or driving. This European formulation has been used on that continent with great success for many years. Each capsule contains 5,850 I.U. (International Units) of Vitamin A and Beta-Carrotene in an oil solution to maximize its conversion to Viatmin A that the body can use.

Juices for Night Blindness

In addition to carrot juice, a variety of juice blends rich in vitamin A may help alleviate night blindness. From the following blends, chose one which best suits your taste. A pleasant taste will help ensure that you drink the juices regularly. Drink the juice in the amounts provided once a day.

1) Fennel 8 fl. oz.

2) Carrot 8 fl. oz. 6 fl. oz.

3) Watercress 3 fl. oz.
   Parsley 1 fl. oz.
   Carrot 10 fl. oz.

4) Papaya 16 fl. oz.

5) Carrot 8 fl. oz.
   Celery 6 fl. oz.
   Spinach 2 fl. oz.

6) Carrot 8 fl. oz.
   Celery 8 fl. oz.

In normal vision—what we call 20/20 vision—there are no errors of refraction. The light rays travel in parallel lines as they enter the eye. They project an image on the retina at the back of the eye, near the optic nerve. (See top illustration.).

In nearsightedness, or myopia, the light rays converge and become focused before they reach the retina. Because of this convergence, the rays start to diverge and become out of focus by the time they reach the retina. The retina then sends that unfocused message to the brain and a person who is nearsighted sees a blurred image.

The extent of the blurred vision depends upon how far in front of the retina the point of focus falls. It can be quite close to the retina, which would cause only a slight blur, or the point of focus can be rather far in front of it, which would make the person's vision worse. (See the middle ilustration)

In farsightedness—or presbyopia—the light rays fall behind the retina before they come into focus, which also causes blurred vision.

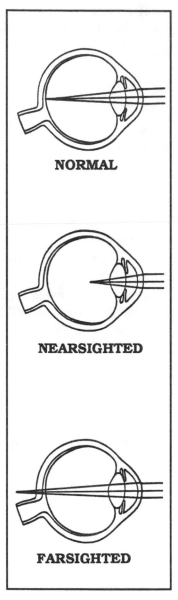

NORMAL

NEARSIGHTED

FARSIGHTED

Chapter 7

Cataracts: Prevention and Treatment

Cataracts are the chief single cause of blindess in the United States. About three million Americans suffer with advanced cases of cataracts. Of everyone living in industrialized Western countries who reaches the age of 60, nearly 60 percent of them have some cataract formation. Moreover, the National Society to Prevent Blindess estimates that in the U.S., about 44 million people aged 40 and over experience some degree of cataract formation.

Cataracts are the best known of the degenerative eye diseases. They result in cloudiness or opacity in one's aging crystalline lenses. As the formation of opacity develops, vision becomes obstructed.

If the opacities are tiny, they cause little difficulty in vision. The areas of cloudiness grow, however, they prevent more and more light from

141

entering the eye. Therefore, the retina receives insufficient light to record an image for the brain to recognized readily.

As the lens becomes progressively cloudy, vision becomes dim and blurry. That's why the person suffering with cataracts requires a brighter light for reading. Or it may be that he will need to bring objects quite close to the eye in order to see them. In other instances, double vision may occur, as in the perception of a street light from a distance. Stationary spots begin to appear in front of the eyes, looking as if they are dust spots on eyeglasses when actually they are opaque spots on the human lens.

Vision may be more accurate for the cataract patient when he performs an activity in twilight. Eventually the cataract becomes obvious to other people by the milky, grayish-white appearance of the person's pupil.

A cataract sufferer loses his sight gradually, over a period of several years. However, there are some cataracts which are caused by a trauma. In these cases, loss of sight is quite rapid, sometimes taking only a few weeks for blindness to set in.

When the formation reaches the stage when the person's sight is obstructed, it is called "mature." Its progression has reached the point where surgery is required. Cataract formation can progress past this point, though, to what doctors call the "hypermature" stage. This is a dangerous point. The eye can very easily become inflamed, thus causing enough pressure upon the optic nerve to cause glaucoma. There is a very real danger in this case of lens rupture.

At that stage, the lens may turn white from the increased swelling. A person with a hypermature cataract that has advanced this far, is for all intents and purposes blind. The most he can distinguish is light or perhaps vague shapes moving in front of him. At this juncture, an emergency operation is imperative to save the eye.

Cataracts, moreover, usually develop in both eyes simultaneously, with one eye generally worsening faster than the other.

The most common cause of this degenerative eye disease is increasing age. This is commonly called the senile cataract and occurs from the lens adding new cell layers to the outside periphery similar to the growth of rings on a tree. These additions change the lens resiliency and clarity. The lens tends to become more rigid and less transparent with time. As we age, all of us are subject to lens rigidity and loss of focus. It's called presbyopia and it's the reason that we need bifocals as we get older. But the decreased transparency which occurs is the cataract itself.

There are other, less common types, known as secondary cataracts, which are not related to aging. Congenital cataract, for instance, is present at birth and is considered a metabolic disease.

Another metabolic condition, galactose cataract, comes from milk sugar accumulation. It results from the person's lack of body enzyme needed to break down this sugar during metabolism. Such a deficiency leads to an absorption of water into the lens and a blocking out of light. Some researchers have found that improved galactose metabolism may be obtained through riboflavin (B2) or orotic acid supplements.

An injury to the eye or lack of suitable protection against occupational hazards, such as excessive heat or radiation exposure, also may result in cataract formation. Moreover, cataract development may be hastened by diabetes, various nutritioinal deficiencies and as an adverse side effect of medication used to treat another disease. Thses are all considered secondary cataracts.

The biochemical process involved in development of this eye condition results from enzyme activities. The enzyme count in the body drops as one ages, especially if less live foods such as sprouts are eaten. Nutritional researchers recommend consumption of adequate amounts of raw vegetables, fruits and grains to prevent cataracts.

Battling Cataracts with Nutrition

One of the best methods for treating cataracts is to prevent them even before they form. Proper eating habits are crucial to maintaining healthy eyes. An increasing number of opthalmologists and physicians recognize that a cataract is not a localized eye problem, but rather a reflection of a condition affecting the entire system.

Research shows that eyes struck by cataracts are deficient in certain nutrients. Scientists have had excellent results in treating this eye condition with certain vitamins and trace minerals. In fact, there are a few advanced ophathamologists who are performing less cataract surgeries and treating their patients through a nutritional approach.

Among the most important of these nutrients is Vitamin C. Abundant medical research now shows that Vitamin C is vital for normal ocular metabolism. Dr. Shambu Varma led a team of researchers at the University of Maryland Medical School, who discovered that Vitamin C occurs within the eye in concentrations 30 to 50 times that found in the circulating blood of the body. In fact, the only area with a higher concentration of this vitamin is the adrenal cortex. Moreover, just prior to cataract formation, the level of Vitamin C in the eye drops

145

dramatically, according to Dr. Varma and his researchers.

Preventive Juice Therapy

Some experts on nutrition suggest that one begins drinking certain juices at an early age, before the onset of cataracts. This will prevent the formation of the opacities, they say. Susan E. Charmine in *The Complete Raw Juice Therapy* (Thorsons Publishers, Inc., 1983), recommends choosing from among the following variety of juice blends.

1) Carrot 10 fl. oz.　　2) Carrot 6 fl. oz.
   Celery 5 fl. oz.　　　　Beet 5 fl. oz.
   Parsley 3 fl. oz.　　　　Cucumber 5 fl. oz.
   Watercress 2 fl. oz.

3) Carrot 10 fl. oz.　　4) Carrot 8 fl. oz.
   Parsley 3 fl. oz.　　　　Watercress 5 fl. oz.
   Spinach 3 fl. oz.　　　　Tomato 7 fl. oz.

How Vitamin C Protects The Lens

Vitamin C is essential to the health of the eye due to its major role in the formation of many of the organ's structures, especially collagen. Moreover,

Vitamin C stimulates and strengthens the immune system, thus helping the eye to avoid infection and diseases, such as cataracts.

But perhaps the most fascinating role Vitamin C plays is in the protection of a certain group of proteins from oxidation which keeps the lens transparent. Should this protein group be destroyed, the lens grows cloudy.

Light seems to be the double-edged sword to the eyes. Because the lens of the eye is transparent, this allows the entrance of light—which is essential for vision. But light—especially the ultraviolet rays—is a key ingredient in the generation of a "superoxide radical," a highly unstable substance extremely destructive to all cells of the body—including the human lens. The destructive forces of free radicals, according to some theories, are the cause of the aging process in the human body. Moreover, this particular free radical forms to create two other types—each as equally damaging as the original.

Australian doctors, for example, examined the eyes of more than 100,000 people from remote rural areas scattered all across the country. The doctors compared the incidence of cataracts with zones of average daily sunshine—in effect the amount of ultraviolet radiation.

The study demonstrated convincingly that a "cataract develops earlier in life and also has more severe visual consequences in areas of high ultraviolet radiation." The extensive examination showed that this conclusion was especially true of Australia's aborigines. These people spend the majority of their lives outside or under inadequate shelter in the bright sun.

But Vitamin C can prevent the accumulation of this substance. It, in effect, scavanges the free radicals and renders them ineffective. Extensive testing shows that when Vitamin C is not present in the human eye, cataract formation begins.

High concentrations of Vitamin C are found in the eyes of animals that are active during daylight hours. By contrast those animals which are noctural had almost immeasurable amounts of the nutrient.

Supplementation of your diet with Vitamin C tablets may be an excellent preventive measure against cataract formation. One of the best formulas available is Vitamin C with Bioflavonoids, which many formulas neglect to add, are essential to activating the nutrient to its full potential.

While Vitamin C can prevent the damaging effects of light upon the eyes, it has been discovered, that too much light can, indeed, destroy Vitamin C. So, what protects this nutrient from ultraviolet rays? The answer is a little polypeptide called glutathione, which has been found to revitalize Vitamin C. As the vitamin is used, glutathione, researchers have found, reactivate the nutrient.

Glutathione is important in the transportation of oxygen, a vital element to the eye. Glutathione, independent studies have found, may also be able to neutralize the effect of environmental pollutants, such as tobacco, upon the body.

Curiously, as the human body ages, the glutathione content in the eye decreases, which may partially explain the reason for senile cataracts.

Riboflavin

Now the question becomes, "What can I do to ensure I have enough glutathione in my system?" Not surprisingly, the answer is still another nutrient—this time Riboflavin, or Vitamin B_2.

Riboflavin is essential for the production of the enzyme—glutathione reductase—which activates glutathione and a second form of the polypeptide. A study conducted by Dr. Syderstriker of the University of Georgia Hospital administered doses of 100 to 300 mg of Riboflavin to 48 early cataract patients who were also found to be deficient in this B vitamin.

149

Within only 48 hours, every patient—without exception—experienced a dramatic imporvement. After nine months, the cataracts of all 48 people were macroscopically indetectable.

According to Earl Mindell, riboflavin is the nation's most common vitamin deficiency. However, please keep in mind that this nutrient also makes the eyes more sensitive to damage from ultraviolet light. It would be wise, therefore, to always wear protective sunglasses when outside in bright light.

In another study, conducted at the Eye Foundation Hospital in Birmingham, Alabama, doctors discovered that 20 percent of a group of cataract patients up to age 50 showed a riboflavin deficiency. Moreover, 34 percent of those beyond the age of 50 lacked this nutrient.

One doctor involved in this study commented, "What is perhaps surprising is the lack of any riboflavin deficiency in our older clinic patients with clear lenses." The possibility that dietary riboflavin supplementation—beyond current recommended levels—may be useful in retarding the formation of senile cataracts is still being heavily investigated.

Selenium, Vitamin E and Cataracts

The trace mineral, selenium, now touted by

many researchers as an antioxidant that may slow the aging process, may also play an equally important role in the prevention of cataracts.

Without selenium, the production of glutathione would be impossible. According to Dr. Alex Duarte, author of *Cataract Breakthrough* (International Institute of Natural Health Sciences, Inc., Huntington Beach, California, 1982), a safe dosage of selenium is about 300 to 400 micrograms daily. He cautions that selenium is toxic when taken in amounts greater than these in the organic form, which incidentally, is the most effective form.

Vitamin E is also an important nutrient in cataract prevention. This vitamin, also considered by specialists in aging research to have antioxidant value, has been proven effective in preventing cataracts in the eyes of rabbits. Researchers at the Mount Sinai School of Medicine, led by Kailash C. Bhuyan, M.D., artifically induced cataracts in the animals, then administered Vitamin E intravenously.

The promising results excited the researchers. In rabbits with early cataract formation, the study demonstrated that the VItamin E arrested and even reversed the eye disease in about half of the animals.

Moreover, the combination of selenium and Vitamin E produces a synergistic effect. This means their value when taken together is highly increased then when either is taken separately.

Another synergistic effect seems to occur when Vitamin E and tryptophan, an amino acid, are administered together. George E. Bunce and John L. Hess, of Virginia Polytechnic Institute and State University, demonstrated that simultaneous deficiencies of the two nutrients in pregnant rats resulted in cataract formation in their offspring. In fact, nearly a third the infants born to the double-deficient mothers developed cloudy spots on their lenses in less than a month. The high incidence rate was not experienced, however, among rats who were lacking only Vitamin E or only tryptophan.

Bioflavonoids

Still another nutrient plays an important role in preventing cataracts which have formed in diabetics. Those suffering with diabetes experience cataract formation at an earlier age than non-diabetics. Moreover, the eye condition progresses more rapidly than in others.

The diabetic experiences an increase in sugar—specifically, glucose—which diffuses into the lens and forces its metabolism to create larger amounts of a sugar alcohol called sorbitol.

Sorbitol then forces an influx of water into the lens, distending the fibers and causing swelling. It is this swelling, by the way, which causes the rapid fluctuations in eyesight for diabetics.

Bioflavonoids, however, may be able to help inhibit the cataracts in diabetics. According to extensive research conducted by Dr. Varma, Dr. I. Mikuni and Dr. J.H. Kinoshita, this vitamin group has impeded formation of the cloudy lens in experiments.

The most effective bioflavonoids are quercetin, quercitrin and myricitrin. These worked by inhibiting the action of the enzyme aldose reductase.

Researchers have tested the effects of quercitrin, the most potent of the trio, on diabetic animals. The scientists chose a South American rodet, called the degu, because it is highly susceptible to the action of aldose reductase. The animal usually develops cataracts less than two weeks following the onset of diabetes.

The group of rodents not given quercitrin developed cataracts within the normal pattern, about 12 days after contracting diabetes. Those administered the bioflavonoid, however, did not expereince cataract formation until 25 days after the onset of the disease, even though the levels of sugar in their blood were about the same as in the other group.

153

The scientists concluded that their study "reveals for the first time" that the inhibition of aldose redactose, not only leads to a decrease in the sorbitol accumulation in the lens, but also impedes the cataractous process. They concluded further that "the cataract formation in diabetics may thus be at least delayed, if not prevented" because of this research.

No daily allowance has been established for bioflavonoids. Most nutritionists agree, though, that for every 500 mg of Vitamin C one takes, he should also take 100 mg of bioflavonoids.

Excellent natural sources of bioflavonoids include citrus fruits, grapes, plums, apricots, currants, blackberries, cherries, green peppers and buckwheat. There is about ten times greater concentrations of bioflvonoids in fresh fruit than in its juice.

Many Vitamin C supplements also contain bioflavonoids, so check your tablets. If the formula you use doesn't contain these nutrients, then consider switching to one that does.

An excellent choice is Vitamin C with Bioflavonoids, available through better health food stores.

The Sun and Cataracts

The sun, indeed, can hasten the development of cataracts according the *New England Journal of Medicine.* The Dec 1, 1988 issue contained a study confirming what doctors and scientists have long suspected: Prolonged exposure to the sun raises a person's risk of developing cataracts.

The research focused on 838 Chesapeake Bay waterman (fishermen, oystermen and crabber) demonstrating that those who do not shield themsleves from the sun run more than three times the risk of developing cataracts than do people who spend a lot of time indoors.

"If there is enough sunshine to make you get a sunburn, then you should really be protecting your eyes," said Dr. Hugh Taylor, associate professor of ophthalmology at Johns Hopkins Wilmer Eye Institute. He was also principal investigator in the study.

Specifically, the study found a link between the sun's ultraviolet B rays, one of two bands of ultraviolet radiation which reaches the Earth, and the formation of cataracts.

The sun has already been implicated in the development of skin cancer and doctors currently suggest protective wear to avoid the dangers of ultraviolet radiation.

Dr. Taylor offered several suggestions to reduce one's exposure to these rays when outside.

155

The Sun and Cataracts (con't)

1)   Wear hats.

Wide brimmed hats are especially good because they block more of the rays from hitting your face.

2)   Wear Sunglasses.

Those glasses with special ultraviolet filters can prevent virtually any radiation from reaching the eyes, but inexpensive sunglasses also help block the rays. Even regular untinted lenses can cut exposure by almost 90 percent and drastically reduce your chances of developing cataracts.

"If we adopt methods of protection to delay formation of cataracts by even 10 years," Dr. Taylor observed, "we could reduce the amount of cataract surgery by 40 percent."

Stress As a Cause of Cataracts

Stress has been shown to interfere with the body's circulatory system, inhibiting the flow of nutrients to the eyes. Stress can also impede the proper lymph flow which provides for drainage and the elimination of the body's toxins to allow the absoprtion of the cataracts.

156

Joan T., for example, discovered that her cataracts were due to stress. She had been recently widowed. During the 40 years of marriage, she had relied greatly upon her husband for answers to many major and minor problems.

Now that he was no longer alive, she was forced into situations where she had to make her own decisions. She barely tolerated this and had a great deal of trouble adjusting to it.

About a year after her husband's death, Joan's eyesight began to dim. Her doctor diagnosed the condition as cataracts and explained that surgery would be an unavoidable fact.

She sought a second opinion upon the urging of a friend. The other doctor had taken a full history and learned of her new found—but unwanted—independence. After a thorough examination, he said what Joan was probably experiencing was stress-induced cataracts.

Gradually, she began to cope with her widowhood and felt much more secure with her new life. Her eye condition, too, slowly improved until it completely disappeared.

Many doctors recommend relaxation techniques for those with cataracts. One professional has used the Bates System of eye exercises for many years and without exception every cataract patient had

157

suffered from some type of prolonged stress or sudden shock and was helped by the system.

Dr. William H. Bates was a New York ophthalmologist who in the 1940s devised a series of exercises after extensive research into vision problems. (For more information and several eye relaxation techniques, turn to page 201.)

Another therapist boasts of a 90 percent success rate with the Bates System, with the following results achieved:

1) Cataracts stopped developing.
2) Cataracts were reduced and vision improved on a continuing basis.
3). In cases where surgery had been advised, it was no longer needed.
4) Patients learned to relax which helped to reverse the condition.

If you are under a lot of stress, you might want to consider vitamin supplements. The B-complex family of vitamins are an excellent, natural way to soothe your ragged nerves and perhaps save your eyesight.

According to nutritionists, the B-Complex vitamins favorably affect your central nervous system.

An excellent, all-natural formula is B-complex Plus, especially developed to create physical and mental energy.

Herbal Remedies for Cataracts

Through the ages, cataracts have been treated with herbs. Today, some herbalists still use a few of the plants to help relieve this condition.

The Greater Celandine, for example, has historically been associated with the treatment of this condition. In medieval times, juice from the Greater Celandinc was used as eye drops for the removal of the clouds on the lens.

Today, herbalists say the juice of this slender plant, when applied to the outside of the eyelid, may gradually fade cataracts and spots on the cornea. Experts emphasize, however, the juice should not be dropped directly into the eye.

Instructions
Greater Celandine

Preparation: Take entire stalk, including the flower. Wash gently over cold running water. Place wet plant in the juice extractor.

Frequency of Use: Apply to outer eyelids several times daily.

Note: The juice will stay fresh for up to six months, if refrigerated.

159

Experts also note that a steam bath for the eyes, made of a blend of herbs, including Chamomile, and Eyebright, has helped cataract patients. This is the same steam bath which we mention for the glaucoma patient. The instructions are on page 189.

Another special combination of herbs, called Samst's Swedish Bitters, is all but unknown in the United States. It's popular in Europe for its powers of curing and alleviating the symptoms of a variety of ailments, including cataracts.

When brushed across the eyelids, Swedish Bitters is said to be an effective treatment for cataracts. It should noted, though, that the herbal blend is highly astringent and precautions, such as coating the skin with Calendula ointment, should be taken.

While we provide the instructions for blending Swedish Bitters, it is also available in liquid form from better health food stores.

Swedish Bitters may also help relieve pain, cramps, constiptation and many other health problems. Herbalists also explain that it is an excellent method of cleansing the body, a process which improves your general health.

Instructions
Swedish Bitters

2 g Saffron
5 g Carline Thistle Roots
5 g Myrrh
10 g Aloe (Wormwood Powder may be substituted)
10 g Senna Leaves
10 g Camphor (Natural Chinese Camphor **must**
   be used)
10 g Rhubarb Roots
10 g Zedvoary Roots
10 g Manna
10 g Theriac Venezian
10 g Angelica Roots

Place these herbs into a two-quart glass bottle with one and a half quarts of pure spirits. Cork and allow the mixture to stand in a warm place for two weeks, strain off the liquid and pour into small glass bottles. Keep the blend away from light and tightly corked in a cool place. Shake well before using.

Note: Be sure to use glass and not plastic containers.

Correction of Catracts

Until recently, the only known treatment for cataract correction was the removal of the lens by means of three types of extraction: intracapsular, extracapsular and phacoemulisification. Surrounding the mass of cloudy lens there is a thin layer called the capsule. In intracapsular extraction, the cataract is taken out along with the capsule. In extracapsular surgery, the posterior capsule is left in place while the cataract is removed. And in phacoemulsification, the posterior capsule is left intact while an ultrasonic needle emulsifies and sucks out the cataract.

About three months after any of these operations, corrective lenses—either eyeglasses or contacts—are fitted to the eye.

About 95 percent of all cataracts are operable. Certain complications are common to all types of surgery, but the chances of those complications developing depend upon the type of surgery performed.

Most eye surgeons are using the extracapsular type of extraction when they remove a cataract, because it seems to reduce the incidence of such complications as retinal detachment, infection, and swelling of the macula (the area of most distinct vision of the retina).

Surgery is most often performed in the hospital with a local anesthetic injected under the eyelid of the patient, just as a dentist injects it under the tooth before performing any prcedure. This method is perferred, because it is much safer than a general anesthesia. This means that the patient is awake during the operation, but feels no pain. The patients will stay in the hospital about three or four days.

The operation takes only about half an hour. The surgeon makes an opening in the upper part of the eye where the cornea is clear, joining the white sclera. With a pair of forceps, a suction cup, or even a freezing probe, he can then grasp the cataract and remove it. As one might imagine, this is an extremely delicate operation and requires a considerbly skilled surgeon. Following the removal of the cataract, the incision is closed with stitches.

The eye is patched following the first week of surgery. In most cases, those who undergo this operation are able to care for themselves and do not need assistance with their daily acctivities. If vision in the unoperated eye is poor, however, the person may need help to avoid accidents.

The patch needs to be changed daily whether at home or at the hospital. A metal cup must be worn over the eye which was operated while the person sleeps. This prevents the opening of stitches or scratching of the eye during the night. The doctor will also prescribe eye drops, which in most instances are used three to four times a day, to hasten the healing process.

Eye irritation may last anywhere from three to six weeks and in some extremely sensitive individuals, up to six months following surgery. During this period, the patient should be making frequent trips to the surgeon to ensure no complications develop.

According to George C. Thorsten, M.D., those who have undergone cataract surgery are more prone to retinal detachment and hemorrhaging. He advises these people to use extreme caution in their daily routine. Avoid any sudden jarring to the head and do not resume heavy, physical labor for at least two months following surgery.

Even, then, Dr. Thorsten notes, that it may be hazardous to place oneself in a position where he may fall. And because vision adjustment is slowed after cataract surgery, patients should not climb ladders due to the very real danger of falling.

Intraocular Lens Implant

A newer, more effective surgical procedure for correction of cataracts is the intraocular lens implant and is inserted in the eye after a cataractous lens is removed. The advantages of this procedure are many, including the relative speed of the operation, which may be performed on an outpatient basis, and the near miraculous restoration of sight in just 24 hours. Here are some questions and answers concerning this procedure.

Q. *What is the Intraocular Lens Implant made of?*

A. The implant is made of polymethylmethacrylate and commonly referred to as PMMA. It is a biologically safe, chemically inert and non-toxic substance which is completely compatible with the eye tissues.

There is no danger to the eye. Degeneration or depolymerization of PMMA has never occurred even after many years of being in the eye. Moreover, the material is strong, lightweight and perfectly transparent. It's perfectly suited as a lens implant.

Q. *Are there different methods of inserting the implant?*

A. Yes. Surgical techniques have perfected two basic methods, the anterior and posterior implants, both of which have been performed with great success.

Of these two, though, surgeons consider the posterior implant the superior. In this procedure the lens is implanted within the posterior chamber itself. This means that it is supported by the patient's own lens capsule which is left in the eye when an extracapsular cataract extraction is performed.

Essentially, the lens is supported by an otherwise nonessential tissue containing no blood vessels, thus greatly reducing the chances of complications. No other area of the body, in fact, provides such a unique medical advantage.

Approximately 80 percent of the implants performed each year in this country are of the posterior variety and the remaining 20 percent are the anterior type.

Q. *Who is candidate for the Implant?*

A. Not every cataract sufferer can undergo this operation, however, the vast majority can. Consult your ophthalmologist to see if your circumstances will allow the intraocular lens implant.

Q. *Can one have the implant if he has already undergone cataract surgery?*

Yes. There is a procedure called the "secondary implant," which allows the person whose natural lenses have been removed to benefit from the implant.

Secondary implants offer patients all the benefits of the primary implant. The patient, following surgery, will experience no distortion, no exaggerated magnification and no malpositioning due to external causes.

Q. *How long does the operation take?*

A. An intraocular lens implant takes about an hour. Vision is restored within 24 hours and after only three to six weeks the operation can usually be pronounced successful.

Q. *How safe is the procedure?*

A. Extremely safe. In 1984, over 700,000 successful implant operations were performed in the United States. It is estimated, moreover, that by 1990, this number will have jumped to over 800,000.

As evidence of the growing popularity and success of the procedure consider these statistics. In 1981, only about 20 percent of all cataract operations were intraocular implants; by 1984, the number had risen to nearly 80 percent.

Q. *Can someone be too old for the implant operation?*

A. No, under normal circumstances, age presents no problem with the lens implant. Successful operations have been performed on individuals who were over 90 years old.

Q. *When should I have an Intraocular Lens Implant?*

A. In the past, patients had to wait until the cataract "matured" before any surgery could be performed. In effect, this means the perrson had to wait until he was practically blind before anything could be done. And the process of slowly experiencing blindness is terrifying.

Fortunately, people need not go through that waiting period today. Intraocular lens implants can be performed with complete success at much earlier stages before the cataract has matured. Very often, the implant can be inserted immediately folowing the confirming diagnosis.

Q. *What will vision be like after an intraocular lens implant?*

A. With this procedure, patients virtually regain normal vision. They have full peripheral vision. Problems with magnifications of objects and depth perception, which have previously bothered some cataract patients in other forms of surgery, are not a problem after this procedure.

Q. *Will daily activities be restricted after the implant?*

A. Very little restrcition is placed upon the implant recipient. For the first three weeks, one should use his own discretion and heavy physical exertion is discouraged.

The patient will be required to wear an eye shield while he sleeps for two weeks following the surgery.

Once the implant has healed, activities can be resumed as before.

Q. *What "famous" people have had the implant?*

A. One cannot tell by looking at a person whether he has had an implant, so it's hard to say. But two celebrities who have undergone the procedure are actor Robert Young and actress Hedy Lamarr.

After the Implant

A person who receives an implant should expect some retrictions upon his activities. His doctor will probably advise that he avoid heavy lifting. While he may bend over to pick up light objects, for example, shoes and books, avoid bending over to pick up anything much heavier, most doctors recommend.

The implant recipient is not restricted in any reading activity, though. Sewing or watching television will not cause any strain to the eye either. And one may look down without any fear. Care should be taken when one walks, to avoid stumbling over steps or curbs.

Depth perception may be slightly abnormal initially, so if you drive a car, use special caution. One should drive, however, only if your unoperated eye is strong enough. Vision in the eye with the implant may be a little cloudy and slightly out of focus immediately following surgery.

The doctor will give the implant recipient a metal guard to be worn at night for two weeks following surgery. With this guard, the person can sleep on either side of body without worry.

Some people are sensitive to light immediately following the implant procedure. The light is not harmful to the eye. It may be more comfortable, for several weeks, though, to wear sunglasses when in bright light.

It is extremely important that the implant recipient avoid direct pressure upon the eye. He should not rub it. He will naturally feel as if there is a foreign material in it. It may also secrete mucus and water. Gently wipe this discharge with moist cottonballs, but do not apply pressure to the eye.

Cataract Surgery: Conditions That May Complicate It

With any of the three surgical procedures for cataract removal--intracapsular, extracapusular or phacoemulsification, there are several existing eye conditions which may complicate the operation. These are listed below. If you have any of these conditions,

---

Cataract Surgery: (Con't)

please discuss them fully with your surgeon before the operation.

Myopia—The danger for a person who is nearsighted is that the thinned retina may detach sometime following the operation, especially if the vitreous jelly is lost during the procedure. The safest of the opertions in this case is the extracapsular because the posterior capsule is left intact, thus preventing the jelly from moving forward.

If the retina does not become detached, the thinning may result in a significant chance the operation may not, ultimately, be successful. This is certainly the case if one has had a retinal detachment prior to the cataract operation. The odds are greatly increased that the retina will detach once more.

Glaucoma—Cataract surgery for a glaucoma sufferer is difficult because the pupils of his eyes are constricted by the eyedrops which control the pressure of the disease. For a successful operation, the pupils must be dilated, or enlarged. Very often, this is almost impossible to do after years of eye drop use. The surgeon must operate, therefore, through a smaller pupil than normal and this may give rise to complications.

It is extremely important, then, for the doctor who is performing the surgery to be experienced with these particular circumstances. Curiously, after the cataract operation, the pressure from the glaucoma

Cataract Surgery: (Con't)

may be relieved, because the surgery has enlarged the drainage areas for the fluid.

Diabetes—After 15 or 20 years from the onset of Type I diabetes—that which affects a person in his adolescent or early adulthood—a degeneration appears in the retina, regardless of whether medication is taken. Called diabetic retinopathy (see page 133, for more information on this condition), its symptoms are hemorrhaging and leakage of fluid in the nerve areas of the retina. Cataract surgery, in this case, may not be able to restore vision as well as in non-diabetic persons, but there will be a reduction in the patient's central vision.

Macular Dengeneration—This condition is basically a hardening of the arteries in the back of the eye. Cataract surgery can leave a person suffering from this with little or no central vision or the lack of ability to read print. Usually, macular degeneration strikes an individual at around 70 years of age or older, but it can affect younger people as well. To test to see if you suffer from this, use the Amsler grid on page 122.

Bleeding Tendencies—If a patient has a tendency to bleed more than normal, cataract surgery may cause hemorrhaging during and after the surgery.

Cataracts Natural Prevention And Treatment Guide	
Vitamins and Minerals	*What They Do*
B-Complex	Favorably works on the central nervous system during times of stress, which may prompt some cataract formations.
Riboflavin (B2)	Essential for the production of enzymes which activate substances protecting the lens from ultraviolet light, a major cause of cataracts.
Vitamin C	Vital to normal ocular metabolism. Important in the formaion of collagen and in strengthening the immune system.
Bioflavonoids	May be especially helpful in preventing cataracts in diabetics.
Vitamin E	May be effective in preventing cataracts. When taken with selenium creates a synergistic effect.
Selenium	Important to the production of glutathione, which protects the eye from ultraviolet light. When taken with Vitamin E may cause a synligistic effect.
Tryptophan	May prevent cataract formation when taken with Vitamin E, thus creating a synergistic effect.

Cataracts Natural Prevention And Treatment Guide (con't)

Herbal Remedies

Greater Celadine Ointment

Herbal Steam Bath

(Eyebright, Valerian, Vervian, Elder

Flowers and Chamomile)

Samst's Swedish Bitters Ointment

Bates Exercise System

Promotes relaxation and use of eyes. Some therapists produce excellent results with cataract patients. See page 201 for some exercises.

174

Chapter 8

Glaucoma: The Silent Eye Condition

Glaucoma has been compared to a thief in the night, sneaking up on a person and stealing his vision. Indeed, this is a very apt description, for unlike just about every other eye disorder, glaucoma provides us with no clues of its existence—until it's too late.

This symptomless condition, which is characterized by an increasing pressure within the eyeball, affects some two million Americans. Of these, approximately *25 percent don't even know they have the condition.* About 600,000 people in the U.S. are blind today because of this condition.

Most tragic of all is that the most common form of glaucoma which accounts for about 90 percent of the cases—causes irreversible permanent blindness.

However, when it is diagnoseed early and treated properly, loss of vision can almost always be prevented

What Causes Glaucoma?

Glaucoma is related to the inability of the aqueous humor, which is constantly circulating in the eyes, to drain properly. Aqueous humor is important because it is the eye's supplier of essential nutrients, the remover of waste products. It also assists the cornea in maintaining its proper curvature and shape.

Aqueous humor should drain out of the eye through the Canal of Schlemm, and thus, a constant pressure is always maintained. However, if for any reason, this Canal is blocked, pressure builds and may slowly deform the opitc nerve, while gradually changing the shape of the optic nerve head. This is the point where it joins the retina.

Eventually the nerve head looks more like a deepening cup. Not only is there nerve head damage externally, but the nerve fibers inside the head are continuously atrophying and dying due to this pressure.

As the glaucoma progresses and the cupping

becomes deeper, blind spots develop in certain areas of the patient's vision.

Usually peripheral vision is the first to diminish, since the nerve fibers which control it suffer the initial damage. Most glaucoma patients are unaware of this development, though, until poritons of their central vision also deteriorate.

A tragic example of this deterioration of side vision concerns a chauffeur, who suddenly became involved in several automobile accidents within a short period of time. His vision was checked and no problems could be found.

Shortly after the examination, he was involved in another accident, in which his automobile struck a young child on a bicycle. The child came from one side, and the driver could not see him. It was after this accident that the driver's side vision was tested. He had no peripheral vision and did not even see the young child unitl he had hit him. The loss of side vision, it was determined, was due to glaucoma.

It is this loss of vision which most often brings a person to an eye specialist, explained Dr. Fritz Hollwich, M.D., of Munster, West Germany. By that time, though, the disease is already in its later stages. Dr. Hollwich estimated that it takes from five to eight years of glaucoma pressure before

177

visual loss is apparent.

Who Gets Glaucoma?

Glaucoma is mainly a disease of the middle aged and older person. It is rarely found in people younger than 35 years of age and affects about two out of every hundred persons over 40. Those at higher risk include people who have diabetes, hardening of the arteries or anemia. Blacks are at a higher risk than the general population as well as those with a family history of glaucoma.

Glaucoma Symptoms

While it is true that glaucoma is a symptomless disease in its early stages, there are signs as the condition progresses. Signals which indicate a person has an advanced state of glaucoma include:

1) Blurred vision and seing rainbow rings around lights— giving them a halo appearance.

2) Seeing halo lights around other bright objects, such as pieces of reflecting metal.

3) Gradual loss of peripheral vision which eventually feels as if you're viewing the world through a tunnel.

4) Inability to adjust to darkened rooms.

5) Need for brighter light to read, sew or to perform other close work.

6) Difficulty in focusing on close work.

7) Difficulty with night driving.

8) Changing eyeglass prescriptions frequently without being able to see better.

9) Severe eye pain with redness and hardness of the eyeball.

Types of Glaucoma

Glaucoma comes in over 30 different forms including the rare cases of infant and childhood galucoma and the more common types which affect older people.

There are many causes for the increased pressure on the eye, including injury, cataracts or inflammation. In some instances, treatment with steroids or other drugs can prompt glaucoma.

The majority of adult cases, though, fall into two categories—chronic, also called open angle and acute, or closed angle.

Acute glaucoma is rare, and may cause vision loss within hours. Fortunatley, the acute version is preceded by a host of symptoms, including blurred vision, colored rings or halos around lights as well as severe eye pain and redness.

Chronic glaucoma—the type almost 90 percent

of those afflicted with the condition have—gives no such advance warning.

Glaucoma Testing

Most eye specialists recommend that everyone over the age of 40 receive a screening for eye pressure at least once every two years. Those at higher risk, such as diabetics or anemics, should be screened more often.

There are sveral methods of detecting increased eye pressure. The method used most often is the Schiotz tonometer. With the person lying on his back, the hand-sized tonometer is placed directly on the front surface of the eye after anesthetic drops have been used.

This instrument is able to indent the cornea through the use of a tiny weighted plunger which is measured on a scale by a simple lever arm indicator. The tonometer is subject to occasional error, though, which is why a newer, high-tech version is now gaining prominence.

It is the Goldman applantation tonometer and is mounted on a slit lamp. Like the Schiotz tonometer, anesthetic drops are applied to the eye. The person is instructed to rest his forehead firmly againt a bar on the slit lamp and to remain as still as possible.

A blue filter is placed in front of the tonometer's light beam and the physician aligns the device with the eye to be examined. The doctor, by moving the entire apparatus, is able to slowly bring the tonometer in direct contact with the cornea. When it has reached the point of clear focus, a pair of bright yellow-green semi-circular arcs appear.

By manipulating the tonometer, he is able to overlap these arcs and then reads the pressure from a scale on the instrument. The process is then performed on the other eye. It is repeated several times on each eye to ensure an accurate reading.

The third device used for glaucoma detection is the "air puff" tonometer, used mainly by technicians and nonmedical eye specialists. It measures eye pressure with a small painless burst of air against the eyeball.

If an ophthalmologist suspects glaucoma, he may want to examine different aspects of the eye's function and structure, beginning with the measurement of "central vision" with a standard eye chart.

Peripheral vision is also inspected for evidence of hidden areas of damage. This is also monitored periodically if a person has glaucoma to make sure that further damage does not occur.

The doctor will then use a goniscopy to examine the interal drainage system of the eye. This is a painless procedure which uses special lenses and lights. This exam indicates whether the increased eye pressure is due to angle closure, which necessitates surgery, or if the drainage system is open.

After all this is done, one more exam is performed—that of the "back of the eye." After dilation of the pupils, the doctor inspects for possible optic nerve damage. He, very often, will be able to correlate the area of visual loss with the appearance of the optic nerve and surrounding tissues.

The blood vessels of the eye and the retina will also be examined to ensure that no additional disease is present which may cause loss of vision.

Nutritional Therapy

The most promising nutritional therapy for glaucoma is Vitamin C. Reports from scientists worldwide testify to Vitamin C's ability to reduce intraocular pressure. Italian ophthalmologist Dr. Michele Virona reported his results at a recent meeting of the Roman Ophthalmological Society.

He and his colleagues administered approximately 7,000 mg of Vitamin C to glaucoma patients five times a day for a total daily dose of

35,000 mg. Within three months all the patients had acquired acceptable levels of intraocular pressure.

Dr. Virona reported that symptoms such as mild stomach discomfort and diarrhea, due to the large doses of the vitamins were only temporary and these side effects disappeared after several days.

Professor G.B. Biett, director of the Eye Clinic at the University of Rome, concurs with his colleagues' findings. Prof. Biett says that Vitamin C therapy for glaucoma is an inexpensive and safe treatment. In fact, he says that the nutritional approach is even safer than eye drops or oral drugs. In many instances Dr. Biett has found that large doses of Vitamin C prevented the patient's sight when drugs and surgery were not effective.

Dr. Fred R. Klennar, M.D., recommends that calcium be taken with the Vitamin C to help minimize any side effects of the large doses.

Rutin, one of the Bioflavonoids, which are also called Vitamin P, has been known to reduce the pressure of glaucoma, recent research indicates.

Bioflavonoids are found naturally along with Vitamin C in foods and their concentration are particularly high in the skins and rinds of many fruits.

In one trial of 26 patients who were given rutin, a drop in intraocular pressure was noted in 17 people. They were given 20 mg of the Bioflavonoids three times daily.

According to nutritionists other good sources of rutin include buckwheat and rose hips. A suggested supplemental dose is 20 mg.

A good supplement, which includes both the Vitamin C and the rutin, can be found in better health food stores.

Other vitamin deficiencies have also been noted in glaucoma patients, most notably Vitamin A. A study in India demonstrated patients with glaucoma had less Vitamin A in their bodies than those without the condition.

Additionally, Dr. Stanley C. Evenas of Ibadan, Nigeria, in West Africa, found that the incidence of this condition was far more prevelant in West Africa than in Europe. He noted that "in West Africa glaucoma occurs at all age levels from children of eight years upwards."

When given a nutritional supplement which included a large dose of Vitamin A, the West Africans' glaucoma was controlled as effectively as it would have been with conventional therapy.

Some physicians recommend daily doses of 7,500 I.U. (International Units) of Vitamin A for glaucoma patients. If you are planning to take this nutrient, experts also suggest a zinc supplement along with it. The Vitamin A needs zinc in order for it it be used by the eye. Moreover, Vitamin E is also required to prevent toxic by-products of Vitamin A metabolism.

An excellent way to receive more Vitamin A in your diet is through supplementation with Eyewell. This all-natural blend of ingredients provides your eyes with extra Vitamin A which may help prevent glaucoma as well as guarding against other eye problems, including night blindness, eye fatigue and sensitivity to reading, driving or watching television.

Other deficiencies noted in glaucoma patients include riboflavin and manganese. Doctors suggest daily doses of 10 mg riboflavin and 40 mg manganese for glaucoma patients.

Stress As A Factor

Some studies show that the more stressful a person is the more prone he is to develop glaucoma. Why this should be, scientists can't say. But supplements of the B complex vitamins may be helpful in these cases, say nutritionists. This group of vitamins helps to minimize the effects of stress on the body. They are nutrients which help repair the central nervous system.

It would be a wise idea if you have glaucoma to schedule plenty of rest periods throughout the day, as well as vacations at regular intervals to avoid excessive stress.

Of course, scheduling "rest periods" into a busy day or regular vacations, is not always possible. In these instances, the negative effects of stress upon the eyes may be reduced by a new European nutritional supplement from Denmark. Recently introduced in the United States, this very special, all-natural formula has already helped thousands of Europeans conquer daily stress and gain new found health.

This vitamin supplement combined with essential rare botanical herbs is discussed in greater detail on page 258.

Six Tips for Glaucoma Patients
There are some things that those afflicted with glaucoma can do to minimize the development of the condition. Here are six suggestions. 1) Quit smoking. Cigarette smoking tends to increase the intraocular pressure of the disease.

Six Tips for
Glaucoma Patients (Con't)

2) Restrict the use of stimulants, such as coffee and tea. Do not drink more than one cup of coffee daily. Switch to herbal teas, which are more relaxing and do not contain caffeine.

3) Do not drink an excessive amount of liquid in a short period of time. Instead of drinking four glasses of fluids at one time, spread this intake in half cup portions over the course of the day.

4) Avoid prolonged periods of darkness, such as watching a movie or television viewing in a darkened room. Keep the use of dark glasses when outdoors to a minimum.

5) Lead as tranquil a life as possible.

6) Watch out for allergies, particularly to drugs, which may intensify your glaucoma. Additionally, be mindful of any new allergies you may acquire as they maybe a reaction to the glaucoma medication. Consult your physician at once if you do develop red, itchy eyes.

To Ease The Pressure
of Glaucoma

In addition to nutritional supplementation and receiving a doctor's attention for your glaucoma, there are several other self-treatments available.

One of these is an *ice cold bath* for your eyes, and is recommended by Dr. Ross Trattler, in his book *Better Health Through Natural Healing* (McGraw-Hill, 1985).

Fill a large basin with ice-cold water, then immerse your eyes in it. Blink rapidly, five to ten times. Take your face out of the water and rest for several moments. Repeat two or three times. Perform this exercise twice daily.

Another treatment is *alternating hot and cold compresses* for the eyes. Apply a hot, moist towel or folded washcloth to your eyes. Allow it to remain for two to three minutes. Then apply a very cold cloth to your eyes for two or three minutes.

Repeat this routine three times, making sure to end with the cold cloth. Perform this exercise twice daily.

Herbal Remedies for Glaucoma

Herbalists recommend several natural alternatives in the prevention and treatment of glaucoma.

Those knowledgeable in herbs suggest a steam bath, made of a blend of herbs, has a positive effect on glaucoma. The instructions follow.

Instructions
Herbal Steam Bath

20 g Eyebright   Boil one pint of
20 g Valerian   white wine and
10 g Vervain   5 teaspoons of
30 g Elder Flowers   these well-mixed
20 g Chamomile   herbs.

With a towel draped over your head and your eyes closed, stand over the mixture and allow the fragrant steam to penetrate your closed lids. Do this for several minutes.

Frequency of Use: Daily

Glaucoma is caused, assert many herbalists, by a problem with the body's kidneys. The next two remedies are said to ease the symptoms of the eye condition by alleviating the kidney problem.

The first is a tea made of an herbal blend which the glaucoma sufferer should drink warm several times daily.

189

Instructions
Herbal-Blend Tea
(For Glaucoma Treatment)

Equal Amounts of:

Stinging Nettle   Speedwell
Calendula   Horsetail

Add 1 Teaspoon:
Swedish Bitters*

Steep the herbs in a quart of boiling water for several minutes, then strain.

Note: Use only freshly-picked herbs.
Frequency of Use: 2-3 Cups Daily

* Instructions for mixing Swedish Bitters are found on page 161. Or pre-mixed liquid Swedish Bitters may be purchased at better health food stores.

The second treatment aimed at healing the ailing kidneys to relieve eye pressure is the *Horsetail Sitz Bath.* It is so beneficial that many people report that pressure is taken off the eyes during the bath itself. When taking the bath, the water should cover the kidney area, but not the heart region. Instructions for the bath follow.

Instructions
Horsetail Herbal Sitz Bath

---

100 g Dried Horsetail Herb
or
1/2 Bucketful Freshly-Picked Horsetail

Preparation: Soak the Horsetail in cold water overnight, making sure the herbs are completely covered. The following day, warm this mixture, then strain. Add the liquid to bath water. Add hot water to the bath as needed to maintain an even temperature. Without drying and wrapped into a bathrobe, one should prespire for one hour in a prewarmed bed.

Note: The sitz bath water should cover your kidney region but not touch your heart area.

Treatments for Glaucoma

Most people with chronic glaucoma can be treated with daily medications. There are several classes of drugs that are designed to increase fluid drainage or to decrease the amount of fluid production, which would regulate the pressure of the eye.

Some of the treatment options are listed below:

1) *Drugs to constrict the pupil.*

This medication, classified as miotics, improves the drainage system and was the most widely used up until recently. *Pilocarpine* is the most common miotic and seldom causes any significant side effects. It is sometimes associated with blurred vision in young people and in older adults with cataracts because it decreases the size of the pupil. Moreover, the smaller pupil may prompt poorer vision in dimly lit rooms.

Pilocarpine drops are used three to four times daily in most cases.

2) *Drugs that dilate the pupil.*

Epinephrine is an eyedrop that reduces the fluid produced by the eye, in addition to slightly improving the drainage system. These drops dilate, or widen the pupil, which may blur vision and may make vision seem brighter than normal.

Epinephrine lasts longer than Pilocarpine, and is only used once or twice daily. Some people, though, develop allergic or irritative reactions to this medication, because it may be absorbed into the circulation. This medication may also prompt heart palpitations or nervousness in some people.

3) *Timolol Maleate*

This drug was approved by the Food and Drug Administration nearly a decade ago and is classified as a "beta blocker." Scientists believe that it is effective because it decreases the production of fluid.

Because it is a beta blocker, people with a history of heart disease, asthma or lung disease, must be extremely careful in its use. If you have any of these conditions and have glaucoma, make sure you tell your eye specialist so he can either prescribe another medication or can monitor you closely.

Most people who use Timolol Maleate, though, experience no significant vision side effects. However, for some, the medication becomes ineffective within several weeks.

4) *Carbonic Anhydrase Inhibitiors*

These drugs decrease fluid production and include *Aceta-zolamide (Diamox)* which is taken orally. This medication is reserved for those who have not responded to eye drops due to the possible adverse side effects of the drug, which include weakness, lethargy, gastrointestinal disturbances and the formation of kidney stones.

5) *Derivative of Coleus Forskohlie*

This drug is only now being developed, but may prove to be the most effective and safest treatment yet. A derivative of the Indian plant Coleus Forskohlie (which is a relative of the multi-colored coleus household plant) this medication works differently than current glaucoma drugs, says Raymond Kosley, Jr. of Hoechst-Roussil Pharmaceuticals, Inc.

"This drug controls (fluid) pressure more directly than others," he noted, which will make it "possible to administer the drug topically, by drops directly into the eye. This means less drug is needed and there is a lessened chance of an adverse side effect."

Glaucoma Surgery

In advanced cases of glaucoma, or in instances where medication produces no improvement, surgery may be required. These methods are not able to reverse the effects of optic nerve destruction which has already occurred. They are, nonetheless, very effective at preventing *further* vision

193

damage.

Until recently, surgery had limited effectiveness because of a lack of precise tools and techniques available. Now, however, the laser beam is rapidly replacing the scalpel.

The majority of physicians welcome the new technology, seeing it as a safe and more effective treatment for glaucoma than conventional surgery. Its main advantage to the patient, is the relative ease associated with laser surgery procedure, which can be performed on an outpatient status at the hospital.

The standard laser treatment, until recently, used the argon laser technique, trabeculoplasty. The eye surgeon aims a 50 micron spot of highly-focused argon energy at the exact location affected by the disease. This burst of energy lasts only one-tenth of a second.

This is done several times along the angle of the person's eye where the aqueous humor is clogged. The energy created by the laser, in effect, "burns" a tiny hole in the eye, which allows for the release of the fluid and alleviates the intraocular pressure.

Many doctors are now using the *Neodymium-Yag* laser. This was first used on ulcer paitnets experiencing hemorrhaging because of the laser's ability to penetrate deeply within the human tissue and stop the bleeding of the large blood vessels. The YAG laser was also used to combat the early stages of bladder cancer. It has proven extremely effective in treating glaucoma.

Beware of Adverse Side Effects

Medication for glaucoma, as for any other medical condition, may produce unwanted side effects in some people.

The beta blocker drugs in eye drop form, of which Timoptin (Timolol) and Beptopten (betaxolol) are two examples, may cause depression, insomnia and even impotence.

Oral beta blocker medication, such as Inderal and Lopressor, may also produce the additional effects of forgetfulness and a slow pulse. They may also aggravate an existing asthma condition.

More serious problems could occur if you are also taking a beta blocker drug for your heart or high blood pressure in addition to one for your glaucoma. The two drugs could interact unfavorably. It is best to advise your ophthalmologist of all the medication you are taking in addition to that for glaucoma.

Side effects may be minimized if you press on the inside of the corner of your eye for 30 seconds to two minutes after placing the drops in your eye. This blocks the tear duct and helps reduce the amount of drug which is absorbed into your body.

Glaucoma Natural Prevention And Treament Guide	
Vitamins and Minerals	*How They Work:*
Vitamin A	Deficiencies of this nutrient have been linked to glaucoma in case studies world-wide.
B-Complex	Helps to reduce the negative effects of stress upon the body, which may be a factor in the development of glaucoma.
Vitamin C	Useful in reducing intraocular pressure.
Manganese	Deficiencies of this mineral have been linked with the occurence of glaucoma.
Rutin (a bio-flavonoid)	May reduce pressure of glaucoma.
Other Natural Methods	
Herb/Vitamin	Special blend of natural ingredients, has beneficial effect on the body. May reduce stress, sometimes the cause of glaucoma.

196

Herbal Remedies

Herbal Steam Bath

(Eyebright, Valerian, Verbain,
Elder FLowers Chamomile)

Herbal Blend Tea

(Stinging Nettle, Calendula, Speedwell,
Horsetail and Swedish Bitters)

Horsetail Herbal Sitz Bath

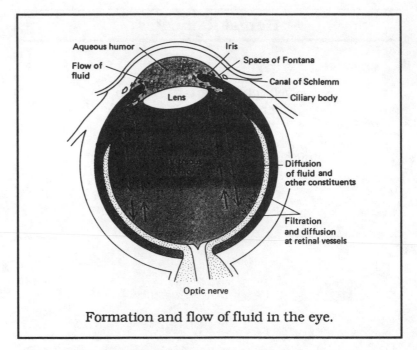

Formation and flow of fluid in the eye.

Glaucoma, one of the most common causes of blindness, is
a disease which increases the intraocular pressure of the eye.
In some cases the pressure can rise as high as 70 mm Hg.
Normally, it should be about 16 mm Hg and in most people
varies from 12 to 20 mm Hg.

Chapter 9

The W.H. Bates Method: Exercises To Improve Vision

Visualize a still pool of water. Now imagine that a half-submerged canoe is rising out of the lake. The canoe appears to bend and curve at the point where it meets the surface of the lake.

The same principle is at work in our eyes. The human eye changes its focus for vision at different distances by altering the curvature of the lens of the eye-at least according to conventional ophthalmic theory.

Light coming into the eye should focus directly on the retina of the eye, but in people who lack perfect vision, it does not do so. In nearsighted people, the light does not quite reach the retina, converging instead somewhere in front of the retina. These myopics must wear glasses for driving or watching movies or television, in other words, for any activity which requires looking into the distance.

Farsighted people (presbyopics) have exactly the opposite situation. For them, light converges behind the retina, making them unable to see things close to them-like the print in a newspaper or phone book. These folks wear reading glasses and when the two problems combine, they are likely candidates for bifocals.

Conventional ophthalmic wisdom states that nearsighted people have long oval-shaped eyeballs while farsighted people have round, fat eyeballs.

Both of these conditions are correctable with eyeglasses or contact lenses, and as is obvious, almost everyone in our society wears one or the other or both.

Eyeglasses and contacts alter the pattern of the light entering the eye. The lenses are ground at a curve which will shorten the light for the farsighted and lengthen the light for the nearsighted, causing it to land directly on the retina.

So, the problem is solved. But is it really? As anyone who has ever worn glasses or contact lenses can tell you, either solution is just a series of problems.

Glasses slide off the nose. They constantly require cleaning and the frames, no matter how minimal, reduce the peripheral vision. Glasses fall out of purses and pockets, are easy to sit on, make us look less than our optimum selves and often times cause headaches when the prescription has not been properly ground or when the eyes change.

As for contact lenses, cosmetic advantages are their big selling point. They can make your brown eyes blue, remove the "lasses with glasses" image and eliminate the peripheral vision problem frames present.

But ask any contact lens wearer, and you will hear a litany of problems. Contact lenses must be boiled or chemically cleaned, they rip, film, stick together and cause the wearer to be one-eyed while a replacement is prepared. They often cause headaches and halos around night lights and in the worst cases, can be responsible for severe eye infections.

In other words, poor vision is a pain in the eyes.

Even its correction, the standard optometric examination, is subject to factors of human error. Do you see the red side or the green side better? Is the upper row or the lower row clearer? True, modern computers have made this process much more accurate, but how many of you have had to return for re-fittings when a pair of glasses or contacts just did not enable you to see properly?

Of course, radial keratotomy, the surgery which we have discussed in this book, is available, but for many of us, surgery is just not a financial or a psychological possibility.

It would seem that there is no solution. Half of the U.S. population wears eyeglasses or contact lenses; 95 percent of Americans over 45 wear corrective lenses for reading and close work. Glasses have been in existence for thousands of years. The Roman writer Pliny notes that the Emperor Nero often used a kind of early monocle to view the gladiatorial games.

Wouldn't it be wonderful if we could get our eyes in shape the same way that we get our bodies in shape-by means of regular exercise?

The good news is that we can get our eyesight into shape, thanks to the pioneering visual work of W.H. Bates, a graduate of Cornell University and an ophthalmologist on the staff of the College of Physicians and Surgeons in New York City. As a staff ophthalmologist at the New York Eye and Ear Infirmary, he examined thousands of eyes a year for several decades using a retinoscope, that ubiquitous machine in the office of every eye specialist, which uses mirrors to focus a beam of light on the eye.

The retinoscope throws light into the pupil of the eye and also casts a shadow at the edge of the pupil. It is the behavior of that shadow which tells doctors the condition of visual acuity in the eye.

Bates' research led him to some startling conclusions. According to Bates, vision adjustments take place in the human eye in the same way that they take place in a camera. Rather than being a permanent condition, vision error is influenced by the ciliary muscles on the outside of the eyeball. Muscles, as we are all aware, can be exercised into shape.

Bates came to his conclusions based on a series of surprising observations. He noted that the eye changes continually over a period of several hours or days, shifting from nearsightedness to farsightedness and back and sometimes landing on perfect vision depending on the time of day that the eyes were examined and on other influential factors.

Stress influenced the acuity of the eye in Bates' tests. He also found that vision changed when the subject coughed, had a cold or fever, was subjected to loud noise, was confused or nervous. Visual range also changes often when we sleep.

In one experiment, Bates examined the eyes of more than a thousand schoolchildren, over half of whom had been tested as having perfect vision. He discovered that when the children were tested at different times and under differing conditions, their eyesight was perfect during some tests and imperfect during others.

The results of these experiments led Bates to the inevitable conclusion that if the accuracy of vision can fluctuate so often and so dramatically, vision problems cannot be permanent. We must have the ability to do something about the accuracy of our vision. "Perfect sight can be obtained only by relaxation," Bates concluded. "The eye with normal sight never *tries* to see."

As a corollary to his research, Bates made some fascinating discoveries and conclusions. He concluded, for example, that our memory and our imagination influence not only what we see but how well we see it. He discovered that schoolchildren have much greater measurable visual accuracy when a word placed on a chalkboard is one with which they are familiar.

He concluded also that we all have illusions of the eyes. We all see colors, sizes, shapes, numbers and locations of objects differently, thus proving that eyesight is influenced by perception.

Thousands of people develop a condition in which they see "flying flies," tiny black specks before the eyes. The specks are non-existent, but nonetheless real to the sufferers. Bates discovered that many of us tend to see complementary colors. If a white piece of chalk appears on a black background, some of us will see it as black on a white background. Of course, we all see blindspots after looking at the sun or looking into the flash of a camera. No spots really appear before our eyes. Instead, our brain is interpreting the experience we have had with blinding light.

Bates research led him to question much of the conventional eye wisdom of the past. (For a complete discussion of this' research and conclusions, read his own book *Better Eyesight Without Glasses*, Henry Holt Inc., 1971, from which much of our information is derived). Bates concluded that it does not hurt the eyes to expose them to fine print or to close work. It does no harm to read in cars or lying down.

He realized that darkness is dangerous to the eyes and always lowers visual acuity if a person's eyes are exposed to the dark for any length of time, a fact that has been borne out by prisoners of war.

Most importantly, Bates came to believe that glasses were, at best, a weak tool to improve the vision and at worst harmful, because they lock the eye into a permanent state of tension in which it can never relax.

Bates' came to believe, as a result of this research that myopia and presbyopia were not the inevitable end results of growing old or of the multiple demands on the eye created by modern society.

Based on that conclusion, the eye doctor developed a series of simple exercises in the 1940s which were designed to relax and strengthen the eyes, thus improving vision. He used these exercises himself, eventually improving his eyesight, over a period of months, to the point where he was able to discard his glasses.

He went on to assist hundreds of people in improving their eyesight, some in as brief and dramatic a time as one day, some over a period of months. Among his more famous patients was Aldous Huxley, noted British author of such classics as *Brave New World.* Huxley was almost blind when he turned to the Bates exercises, and although he was never able to function completely without glasses, the exercises saved Huxley's sight so that he could continue to write. (For the complete story of Huxley's vision recovery read Huxley's own book *The Art of Seeing,* Harper & Row, 1942.)

Here, for you to strengthen your own eyesight, are a sampling of Bates' pioneering techniques. Again, for a more complete understanding of how and why these exercises work, consult Bates' own text *Better Eyesight Without Glasses.*

Palming

Bates discovered that when we focus at the center of the fovea of the eye, the eye automatically achieves perfect vision. He called this principle "central fixation." They eye only achieves central fixation when it is in a perfectly relaxed state. "The vision in the eye *always* becomes normal when the eye looks at a blank surface without trying to see," Bates said.

For that reason, palming provides both the blank surface and the relaxtation necessary to create perfect vision.

Close your eyes, warm your hands, cover your eyes with the palms of your hands, gently blocking out all the light without pressing against the surface of the eyeball. Notice whether you "see" absolute blackness behind your eyes.

Most people whose eyes are under strain are those who do not have perfect vision. They will see kaleidoscopes and colors behind their eyes. Only those with perfect eyesight see absolute black because their optic nerve is not agitate.

If you do not see black, there are several ways to facilitate it. Place a black object at a comfortable distance in front of you and look at it, but stay relaxed. Don't strain your eyes while staring at it. Then, close your eyes and "see" that same black object behind them.

Or you can imagine a small black dot. Allow the dot to grow larger and larger until it fills the space behind your eyes. If the dot does not fill your internal screen with blackness, then imagine deep black fur or the center of a black hole.

Rest this way with your palms over your eyes for several minutes. Do this several times a day. The blackness will grow darker and more absolute as your vision improves.

Palming, in effect, acts as a constructive form of meditation. Exerting any effort in this process will hinder the relaxation which is one of the major purposes of this exercise.

If, indeed, you do see the "black" and nothing else, you have reached the pinnacle of palming. But do not consciously work to reach this effect. With time, it will gradually happen.

If you feel restless while performing this drill— and if you're like many today who are not quite comfortable with doing nothing, you probably will —simply stand up and gently shake out any tension in your body. If your arms get tired while palming, lower them for short time or shake them. You might even want to move them in an easy rhythm. Then continue the exercise.

This exercise is so simple that it can be done almost anywhere—at home, in the office, while a passenger in an automobile or in an airplane.

Palm as often as you can and for as long as you can. Even as little as five minutes of palming in the middle of a hectic work day will refresh you—and your eyes.

Moreover, this exercise and its meditative effects have been known to ease the pain of a headache, especially if it is caused by tension.

If you have any vision defects—nearsightedness or farsightedness—you may want to try palming for 20 minutes in the evening. As we noted, many times these defects are due to the effects of stress.

Lighting

Contrary to the old wives' tales, exposing your eyes to light does not harm them, it actually benefits them. That is of course if you follow precautions and use common sense. You should never look directly into the sun or into an artificial light source. But by exposing your closed eyes to a light source, you relax the muscles, warm the eye and create the proper relaxed atmosphere for perfect vision.

In good weather, always use the sun for the following exercise, but in poor climates a 150-watt light bulb will serve the same purpose.

Sit relxed in a chair outside in the sunshine or six (6) feet from the light bulb. Close your eyes and lift them to the light. Move your head from side to side in a slow, rhythmic movement for three to four minutes.

Restrict your first session of this drill to only one or two minutes and gradually build the time you can light.

Lighting should never be done with a sunlamp, heat lamp, or fluorescent light.

The effects of lighting are many. It may help clear bloodshot eyes and helps to eliminate the occasional itching of the eyes. In fact, the next time you feel like rubbing your itchy eyes—don't. Light them instead. You'll find its much more effective and healthier.

Lighting stimulates the retina, which grows dim and insensitive if it is deprived of an adequate amount of light. When stimulated, the retina transmits images to the brain along one large nerve and eventually along several nerve pathways to the "vision site" at the back of the brain.

These nerves are considered as part of the

brain. Regular use of them sets up reverberations in other brain nerves, according to Bates therapists, in related areas, which actually increase the brain's activities.

Shifting, Swinging, and Flashing

One of Dr. Bates' interesting discoveries was that in normal vision, the eye shifts constantly from side to side or up and down. He found that more than sevently such shifts may take place in a fraction of a second when a patient was reading an eye chart.

The *Snellen Chart*, that descending and shrinking set of letters we have all attempted to read in the eye doctor's office, was the invention of Dutch ophthalmologst Herman Snellen of the Netherlands. It became one of the primary tools Bates used to improve his patients' vision.

He called the Snellen chart an "optimum," that is, something we see clearly and perfectly when we repeat seeing it often enough. A mother's face is an optimum to an infant, for example. The infant will always see her face in perfect focus whereas a stranger's face will be blurred. In the same way, the Snellen chart, when it is a familiar househould object, can improve visual acuity.

211

Bates recommended that every home and class-room should have a Snellen chart hanging on the wall. Persons should stand at a distance of 10, 14 or 20 feet from the chart and devote thirty seconds a day to reading the smallest line on the chart with one eye covered, then the other.

His classroom experiments bore out his belief that this exercise would improve visual acuity. In schools where Snellen charts were placed perma-nently on the classroom wall and where students regularly spent thirty seconds a day reading the bottom line with one eye after the other closed, there was a much lower rate of myopia. Again, this demonstrated Bates' conviction that vision nor-malizes when we look at a blank or familiar surface without straining.

Shifting

Look at any letter on a Snellen chart, then shift to another letter several spaces across on the same line. Shift back and forth between the letters.

Now look at one of the large letters near the top of the chart, then look down at one of the smaller letters. Shift back and forth.

Finally look at a whole Snellen chart hung 3-5 feet away, then shift to one hung 10-20 feet away. Shift back and forth between the two charts.

Swinging

Stand with your feet one foot apart, facing one side of the room. Lift your left heel off the floor, turn your shoulders, head and eyes to the right until your shoulders are parallel with the right wall.

Now do the same motion to the left, raising your right heel. Move your head and eyes gently back and forth with the motion of your shoulders.

In addition to benefiting cases of nearsightedness, farsightedness and crossed eyes, the Swinging exercise, according to Dr. Bates, has also helped relieve several cases of double or multiple vision.

This easy exercise will also increase your circulation and prove to be extremely relaxing. Dr. Marilyn B. Rosenes-Berrett, a Bates therapist and author of *Do You Really Need Glasses*, suggests that Swinging be performed upon rising in the morning—to help one face a long, challenging day—and before retiring for the night. It has been known to help insomniacs sleep.

She advises, that if possible, you perform this exercise while listening to some relaxing music.

It is best to perform the Swing three times daily. Start off with 30 complete swings and increase the amount daily until you are doing 100.

Short Swings

Older people who cannot stand for long periods of time can benefit from a variation of the Swing by performing *Short Swings*, which can be done while sitting.

Sit comfortably in a straight back chair in front of a window. Take your glasses off and allow your hands and arms to loosely hang at your side.

With your nose pointing ahead, keep your eyes open and turn the upper half of your body from side to side. Turn your head with your body. Your arms should be swinging in a free and rhythmical fashion.

After a few swings, look at the top of the window. Imagine a line from the top of the window to the corners of the room. Make sure this line is smooth and flowing. Do not break it. This may take a bit of concentration, so do not get upset if you have trouble doing it at first.

When your eyes pass the window during your swing, allow them to look out it. Look at objects as distant as possible. The change of focus will loosen the eye muscles. Just be sure to keep your vision on the line you traced across the wall.

Perform about 30 of these initially and gradually add more daily until you are performing about 100 swings. As with the regular Swinging exercise, it is best to perform it three times daily.

Lazy Eight Exercises for Relaxation

Lazy Eights when performed slowly and rhythmically, loosen the back of the neck and exert a calming effect on the entire nervous system, explain vision therapists.

This exercise is extremely simple, all you have to do is draw imaginary figure eights with your nose. When you draw large figures, you are relaxing the larger muscles of the eyes. When you draw smaller figure eights, you are allowing the tiny eye muscles to relax.

Performing this exercise also sends more blood to the head, neck and eyes.

The great aspect about Lazy Eights, though, is that they can be done anywhere without anyone noticing you.

To perform this exercise, follow these simple instructions:

Close your eyes. Draw a number eight with your nose, moving your head slowly and smoothly as you do this. Vary the type—draw vertical one, then horizontal ones for several moments. Just remember to move your head slowly and smoothly.

If you tire of drawing eights, try other objects. For example, draw a pie and then cut it into wedges. Or draw wagon wheels and place spokes inside of them.

The only requirement if the *you move your head slowly and evenly.*

Perform this exercise at least three times daily, more if you wish.

Flashing

Rest your eyes for a few minutes, then palm the eyes for a few minutes. Open your eyes for a fraction of a second and look at a letter on your Snellen chart. Now close your eyes. Repeat this opening and closing fifteen to twenty-five times.

Modern Adaptations

The following modern adaptations of Bates' methods are based on the book *Totally Natural Beauty* by Nona Aguilar, published by Rawson Associates in 1977.

Photo Exercise

Cut out several clear magazine photos containing very distinct objects. Try to select magazines in which the paper is not too glossy. Mount these photos on cardboard and place them at the distance where your eyes will see the picture comfortably and clearly.

First look at the photo with each eye covered. Now swing your head from left to right several times. Stop. Look at the figures in the picture in front of you.

Now move your head up and down several times. Stop and again regard the figures in the picture.

Next, hold the photo in your hand and move it closer to you and farther from you, watching the figures in the picture as you do.

Do all of these exercises first with one eye covered, then with the other covered, then with both eyes open. Repeat several times.

Swing Ball Exercise

Using a small, juggling-sized ball, toss the ball in the air from your right hand to your left hand. Let your eyes follow the gentle arc of the ball without permitting them to run ahead of the ball to the opposite hand.

When the ball reaches the left hand, toss it into the air toward the right, following the motion.

Repeat this exercise 25 times and do not let your eyes leave the ball.

Shift Ball Exercises

Again using your fist-sized ball, toss it against the opposite wall so that it bounces against the wall, hits the floor and comes back to you in a triangular pattern.

Once again, you must keep your eyes on the ball, not letting them race ahead to the floor or wall.

Repeat this exercise 25 times.

Hints for Healthier Television Viewing

We all watch too much television. It's almost unavoidable. But it is also unhealthy for the eyes to remain fixed on one object for extended periods of time. So here are some hints, using the Bates vision therapy method, of helping your eyes cope with television viewing or any extended period of gazing.

1) Keep your eyes gliding from one point on the screen to another and then another. The eyes normally shift 80 times per *second* and prolonged staring impedes their movement.

2) Look away from the screen occasionally to

Hints for Healthier
Television Viewing (Con't)

glance around the room for a change of focus.
Look at something on the wall or look at your
watch or the couch.

3) Shut your eyes every so often—you will probably not miss much of the program.

4) Blink frequently while watching television.

Snellen Chart Exercise

For the home which lacks two Snellen charts for
close and distant focusing, this exercise will sub-
situte household objects for the same effect.

Choose several close and distant objects in a
room of the house or outside. The outdoors is a
particularly good choice here because you can
focus on the horizon and then your own fence or on
your neighbor's house and then your children's
swingset.

Look alternately at the distant object then the
near object, repeating and reversing the process
several times.

Don't stare at the objects. Simply let your eyes
move gently and naturally from object to object. Do
this several times daily.

Exercises to Reduce Astigmatism

Astigmatism is caused by tension or pressure on the eyelids or eyeball due to an irregularity in the curvature of the cornea.

Therefore, according to vision therapists who follow the Bates method, relaxation is an important requirement for reducing astigmatism. A useful routine should first begin with palming and lighting drills, then perform the Swinging or Short Swing exercises.

This will relax you and your eyes and prepare you for the following two exercises aimed at easing the shifting of your eyes.

For the first exercise you will need a wire coat hanger and about 12 inch-long pieces of colored tape, get as many different colors as possible.

Bend the hanger in a hoop and wrap the tape, at equal interval, around it.

Hold the hoop broadside at eye level in front of you, about a foot from your face.

With a gentle head motion, guide your eyes clockwise from one piece of tape to the next, until you have circled the hoop three (3) times.

Then close your eyes, recalling mentally the appearance of each individual tape. Circle the hoop in your mind three times.

Repeat the entire procedure going counterclockwise this time.

Another excellent drill that improves astigmatism, Bates adherents say, requires a yardstick and a red marker. A crayon or red pencil will work fine. Again, the idea is to improve the ability of your eyes to change focus.

Mark off the inches of the yardstick with bold red lines. Hold the stick horizontally in front of you at arm's length. Be sure that it is at your eye level.

Smoothly, guide your eyes along each individual inch. Go back and forth several times.

Close your eyes and mentally visualize each red inch mark.

Open your eyes. Move the yardstick to the left while your eyes move to the right. Then move the stick to the right as your eyes smoothly travel to the left.

Now hold the yardstick vertically. Move your head slowly up and down, taking note of each individual inch mark. Do this several times.

Move the yardstick downward, as you move your head upward. Then move the stick up as you move your head down. Repeat several times.

221

Perform these drills at least once a day. In addition, play solitaire and do the eye exercises involving dominoes which are described in the following section for aiding myopia.

How to Remove Spots Before the Eyes

Just about everyone at one time or another complains of seeing spots before their eyes. This phenomonem is especially prevalent among older individuals. In fact, there's even a technical term for those spots—*muscae vaituntes* (flying flies). Most people refer to them as floaters.

The spots are extremely tiny specks which are floating in the eyes' internal fluids. When they appear, try not to look at them, but look past them, keeping your eyes on larger, more important objects. Don't strain your eyes and don't stare.

Bates exercises to help reduce the incidence of these spots include *palming, lighting, swinging and lazy eights.*

Vision Training to Correct Myopia

Begin your vision therapy for the correction of nearsightedness with several minutes of palming and lighting routines. Then place six ordinary dominoes having no more than 12 dots each an inch apart from each other at face level. Sit far enough away from the dominoes so they appear slightly blurred.

Now take your glasses off and relax. Inhale deeply and slowly; exhale deeply and slowly. Open your eyes and allow them to gently wander around the sides, tops and bottoms, of the domino which is located farthest to the left. Don't strain to see the domino dots-just look at the rim. Try to feel that you are looking from the back of your brain where the visual processing occurs.

If the dots are not clear and sharp, close your eyes and visualize the first domino. Imagine it as being sharper and brighter than how you actually saw it.

Imprint that sharp clear image upon your memory. Memory, Bates therapists tell us, is an extremely important part of good vision. Remember, Bates demonstrated that we see familiar objects more clearly than ones which we have never seen before.

Open your eyes and, while keeping the crisp image of the domino in mind, allow your eyes to move once again around the sides of the object. The memorized and projected image will make it more clearly visible.

Repeat the prcedure with the other dominoes.

Each time that one stands out sharply, memorize it immediately and visualize it while your eyes are closed.

When all the dominoes appear clear, open your eyes. Move your chair back a little and repeat the exercise. This may sound as if it would take a long time, but it really doesn't. So don't be frightened of it. If you can spare a half an hour, then you can practice the exercise. If you can spend even more time with this drill, you will observe even faster results. But a half an hour a day will work.

The following day, use playing cards instead of dominoes. Use the numbered spades. Do not use the face cards or the aces.

With clear cellophane tape, place them on a wall at eye level, about one inch apart from each other. Sit far enough away from them so they appear slightly out of focus, just as you did with the dominoes. Repeat the domino exercise with the card, outlining and visualizing them.

Third Day of Training

Substitute a calender on the third day of exercises. Be sure the numbers are large enough to be read at about 10 feet without glasses. Again, the numbers should only be slightly out of focus.

Notice, that in all probability, you should be able to sit a little farther back this time, because of the images you imprinted upon your mind the first two days of practice.

Again, perform the exercise just as you did the dominoes and playing cards. After eight days of alternating the three drills, start your half hour exercise session differently. Place one domino where you can see it perfectly and another where it is slightly blurred. Look back and forth between the two for about 10 minutes. Pause frequently during this drill and concentrate on their rims, rather than on their pattern of dots.

Resume the regular domino exercise for the remainder of your practice time.

Continue this system for at least one month. If you get bored with these objects, try looking at something different, for example magazine pictures, printed signs—any object with an interesting pattern will work.

Supplemental Drills

In addition to the drill, play the card game solitaire whenever you can. This promotes muscular flexibility and is not a game which creates tension, as some games do.

Bates therapists say that by the end of one month most people realize a considerable improvement in their vision. They caution, though, that severe cases of myopia will require a longer period of exercise before improvement will be noticed.

Vision Training for Presbyopia

For those afflicted with presbyopia—the inability of the eye to accomodate at close distances—the exercises to improve myopia will usually help, say vision experts.

In addition to performing those daily, however, add an emphasis on shifting focus from far to near objects and then back again. Other good drills to help ease presbyopia, say the therapists, include juggling, and playing the card game solitaire and ping pong.

Provided below are two more exercises designed to help presbyobics:

Circles

1) Hold a brightly colored ball, Christmas tree ornament, or even a lemon or orange in front of you.

2) Keep your eyes focused on it and then draw circles in the air with it—first small circles and then increasingly larger ones.

    This drill, when performed regularly, will release the eye muscles. Presbyopia is caused

---

Vision Training for Presbyopia (Con't)

by rigid muscles which are not able to focus as easily as they once did.

The Playing Card Drill

Bates therapists say that this drill is extremely helpful for advanced cases of presbyopia.

1) Sit where you can see a picture on a wall some distance from you.

2) Hold a playing card with black numbers (do not use the ace or face cards) at a comfortable reading level, but close enough that the numbers are slightly out of focus.

3) With card in hand, outline with your nose using slight head motions. Shift your eyes to the picture on the wall and outline that in the same manner.

4) Alternate between the card and the picture—outlining each—until you are bored.

5) Then close your eyes and in the same way you outlined the card and picture, "draw" figure eights. Then return to the objects, outlining them.

6) If you can do this exercise for 20 minutes a day, therapists say, improvement will occur. However, even shorter periods of practice will help.

If you follow the Bates exercises faithfully, spending 10 to 15 minutes a day practicing them, you will find that your vision may, indeed, improve.

Bates' patients sometimes also experienced wonderful side effects. Headaches and tension disappeared, memory improved and hobbies which had been nearly or completely abandoned could be taken up again.

But what better side effect could possibly exist than to see perfectly a breathtaking sunset, a beloved face, the distant moon and stars or the clear black words on the page of a book?

For more information on the Bates Method of Eye Exercises, contact the National Center whose address is listed below. They will be able to refer you to a trained visual therapist in your area.

Bates-Corbett Teachers Association
11303 Meadow View Road
El Cajon, California 92020
(714) 440-5224

Chapter 10

Hidden Secrets to Save Your Eyesight

Sound nutrition is important for the proper functioning of all organs of the human body, including the organ of sight, the eye. A lack of certain vitamins can cause the eyes to work at less than their best, just as a lack of iron causes our blood to become less efficient.

The most important vitamin to the health of the eyes is Vitamin A. Its benefits are more far reaching than enabling us to see at night. Prolonged lack of the "eye vitamin" can do irreversible damage to the entire eye. The vitamin is essential for the proper maintenance of the body's moist surfaces, such as the eye.

The first warning sign of a serious deficiency is the drying of the conjunctiva, or the white part of

229

the eye. It loses its natural moisture, as well as its whiteness, and becomes more susceptible to infections.

Uncorrected, the condition next affects the cornea. It, too, will lose its natural moisture and will no longer be smooth. The cornea, additionally, acquires a smoky or milky appearance, giving the person afflicted with this condition the feeling of looking at the world through frosted glasses.

In the final stages of the VItamin A deficiency, the damage goes past the cornea, exposing the interior of the eye and allowing serious infections to set in. The net result is loss of the eye and complete blindness.

As with night blindness, prevention can be relatively simple with the addition of beta-carotene and VItamina A into the diet. In fact, raw carrot juice, an excellent source of beta-carotene, is considered a natural solvent for all ulcerous conditions, such as the cornea experiences in a serious Vitamin A deficiency.

If one medical estimate is accurate, approximately 20 percent of the population is deficient in Vitamin A, although, not to the point, obviously, which would cause severe eye damge. And while many people don't consume enough of the Vitamin A-rich vegetables, there are other reasons why so many of us lack this nutrient.

Vitamin A appears to be highly fragile nutrient. Many ordinary conditions can cause either a decrease in its effectiveness or its destruction. Anyone who works under harsh, glaring lights—especially fluorescent—is a candidate for a mild deficiency. These lights cause the human eye to use up Vitamin A at an accelerated rate. Experts suggest—although at this point they're not sure—that the minute flickerings of the fluorescent causes this consumption. They compare it to the oncoming headlights at night when one is driving. This also causes a large consumption of Vitamin A.

So, even if one receives enough Vitamin A, he may still need a larger intake because of the lighting. It would be wise then, to take a supplement. *Biowell* makes *Eyewell,* which may be the ideal supplement for office workers.

Other causes of rapid usage of Vitamina A include air pollution, excessive television viewing, X-ray treatment, and exposure of the eyes to sun glare, such as that experienced when one skis or surfs.

In addition, Vitamin A can be destroyed if one's liver is not functioning properly, or by alcohol abuse. The use of simple supplements, or home remedies can render Vitamin A ineffective. For example, if one is taking ferrous sulfate—a form of iron—or using mineral oil, some Vitamin A will be destroyed before the body can utilize it.

And if all those conditions weren't enough, here's two more. Any type of infection which one acquires will reduce the nutrient's efficiency, as will one's continued exposure to cold weather. Those who have to work outside during the winter might want to try *Eyewell* also.

Drinking raw carrot juice, then, is a good habit for the overall health of the eye. You can find the instuctions for making the juice on page 138. I. It is also a good habit to munch on fresh carrots as a snack. Don't peel them just scrub them well.

If for some reason, you find carrots difficult to bite, grate the vegetable instead and consume it that way. This is just as effective. As with the juice, though, prepare only the portions you plan on eating immediately, as the natural nutritional strength of the grated carrot weakens as it sits.

Beta-carotene - the product the human body uses to make Vitamin A - is also found in deep orange fruits and vegetables. Good sources include, broccoli, apricots and squash.

It is best to consume fresh sources of Vitamin A, say the experts, rather than relying solely on vitamin supplements. Such supplements expose

232

the body to possible overdoses. While pregnant women's need for vitamins is greater than the rest of the population, as noted in the following chart, medical sources caution that overdoses may produce abnormalities in unborn babies. Doses of 50,000 I.U. daily are considered dangerous.

Recommended Daily Allowances (RDA)	
Vitamin A	
Men	10,000 I.U.
Women	8.000 I.U.
Pregnant Women	12,000 I.U.

If you don't eat enough fruits or vegetables, you can insure you receive enough Vitamin A through a supplement. There are many on the market, but the best are found in good health food outlets.

In fact, smoking tobacco destroys large amounts of the body's reserves of Vitamin B12. A symptom of a B12 deficiency may be difficulty in reading or eyes that tire quickly.

The problem, according to medical professionals, is that the tar and nicotine decompose the eye's myeline sheaths that protect the nerve endings. Smokers sometimes suffer from *smoker's amblyo-*

pia. Smokers who lack enough Vitamin B12 may also complain of frequent headaches and black-outs, as well as difficulty in distinguishing the colors green and red. Moreover, if a person's finger-tips turn cold after his first morning cigarette, it is likely he is deficient in B12.

Merely curtailing cigarette smoking often relieves the symptoms if the deficiency is not extremely severe. Also, if doses of the vitamin are taken before the deficiency has progressed considerably complete recovery is almost certain, say experts.

A deficiency of Thiamin, sometimes referred to as Vitamin B1, moreover, may cause pain behind the eye. With a more serious lack of the vitamin, paralysis of the eye muscle may occur.

The B vitamins also are credited with relieving chronic watery eyes, blood-shot eyes, and aiding in the eye's sensitivity to light.

These vitamins are found naturally in a wide variety of foods, including whole grains, unpolished brown rice, legumes, nuts, green vegetables, poultry, eggs, fruits, fish and meat. Additionally, brewer's yeast is a great source of the B-Complex vitamins.

Despite the seemingly relative abundance of these nutrients, many people do not receive enough of the vitamins in their daily diet. In these instances, a supplement is suggested. One of the best is B-Complex Plus, which provides an excellent supplemental source in a natural formula.

Vitamin D and Calcium

If you're a female and concerned about the possible onset of osteoporosis, you're probably conscious of your Vitamin D and calcium intake. But chances are you didn't realize you may very well be helping your eyes by taking these nutrients.

Dr. Arthur Knapp, a New York City ophthalmologist, has successfully treated a number of eye disorders—including nearsightedness—using these two nutrients. In several cases, those who were nearsighted reported that their visual acuity had *actually doubled.*

Many of those involved in the testing reported a stabilization of their vision which was, prior to the treatment, been declining at an alarming rate.

Other eye ailments which responded to the calcium and Vitamin D treatment of Dr. Kanpp's included keratoconus—a protusion of the cornea—cataracts, retinitis pigmentosa, detached retina and glaucoma.

235

Herbal Aids for Healthy Eyes

In an age that requires increasingly more complicated technology to treat the body's physical ailments, many people are surprised by the almost magical powers herbs possess in alleviating aches and pains.

Herbs, some of which have been used since the times of the ancient Eqyptians, can be effective treatments for the eyes. And the treatment can take many forms-washes, compresses, even teas to drink regularly. We've already discussed a steam bath of a special blend of herbs (see page 190) and Swedish Bitters applied to the eyelids (see page 160) are effective treatments for cataracts. There are several other herbs, long known to other generations, that can ease eye problems.

Yarrow Tea, when taken regularly, aids in relieving the pain behind the eyes and eliminates excessive tearing. This tall herb carries finely-toothed leaves and its flowers are white, pale pink or lavendar, closely resembling tiny clusters of daisies.

Instructions Yarrow Tea	
Preparation	Pour 6 ounces of freshly boiled water over 1 heaping teaspoon of minced Yarrow. Allow the covered mixture to steep for 3-4 minutes. Strain. Drink unsweetened.
Frequency of use	1-2 cups daily

We have already been introduced to the herb *Chamomile* as a wash for relief from conjunctivitis. This herb can also be applied in a compress form (directions on page 127), reducing eye pain and relieving the unattractive bags under the eyes.

A compress made of the *Mallow* herb is also an effective treatment for strained and tired eyes. As a mild wash, the herb opens clogged tear ducts.

The herb has a long slender stem, with rounded, toothed leaves and small pale pink or purple flowers.

Instructions Mallow	
Preparation as a Wash	Soak 1 heaping teaspoon over- night in 6 ounces cold, fresh water. Strain. Warm slightly before using.
Frequency of Use	Daily
Preparation as a Compress	Prepare as directed above. Then wet a cottonball or gauze with the mixture and apply to the eyelids.
Freqency Of Use	Daily
Note	Mallow should never be heated. Heat destroys the medicinal properties of the herb.

Calamus, or *Sweet Flag*, is also an effective herb in strengthening tired and weak eyes. The herb grows wild in marshes and on the banks of ponds and lakes. Its leaves resemble swords. Use of the herb's root as a juice is recommended by herbalists as an external application to the eyelids.

Instructions
Calamus Root Juice

Preparation	Clean the fresh root thoroughly, ensuring all clinging soil is cleaned. Still wet, place in a juicer.
Use	Dip the juice in a cotton pad, and spread it over the eyelids. Allow it to remain for several minutes. Rinse with cool water.
Frequency of Use	Can be repeated several times throughout the day.

Homeopathic Remedies

The following is a list of remedies recommended by homeopathic specialists to aid in the healing of eye infections and inflammation:

1. *Euphrasia 6X*—Aids in the treatment of excessive watering of the eyes and the associated burning.

2. *Physostigma 6X*—Relieves irritability due to excessive use; spasms in the ciliary muscles; twitching; intolerance to light; astigmatism.

239

3. *Graphites 30X*—Relieves red, swollen eyelids and eczema of the lids.

4. *Ruta Graveolena 30X*—Relieves pain from overuse of eyes.

5. *Silicea 30X*—Relieves swelling of the tear duct; pus in eyes and styes.

6. *Cyclamen 30X*—Treats double vision, sparks before the eyes.

7. *Jaborandi 30X*—Treats nearsightedness; eyestrain; white spots.

8. *Nitric Acid 30X*— Relieves the feeling of a splinter in the eye.

9. *Spigelium 30X*—Relieves the stabbing pain in the eye.

The following list of homeopathic recommendations treats injuries to the eye:

1. *Aconite 6X*—Heals injuries from overexposure to dry, cold winds, reflection from snow.

2. *Arnica 6X*—Treatment of black eyes and bruised soreness from close work or eye strain from sightseeing.

3. *Belladonna 6X*—Relieves throbbing pain; especially effective when "the cold settles in the eye."

4. *Hamamelia 6X*—Relieves painful weakness; hastens interocular hemorrhage absoprtion.

5. *Lachesis M-Potency*—Treats defective vision after severe illness.

6. *Ledum 30X*—Relieves bruises, insect bites.

Exercise and The Eye

We all know the benefits of exercise - a healthy heart, strong muscles, increased flexibility and healthy eyes.

Healthy eyes? It just might be so. One of the benefits of exercise is improved circulation. The more efficiently the body is able to pump blood to its cells and tissues, the greater the amount of the essential nutrients are received to ensure their proper functioning. Many of the ills of the eyes, such as cataracts and night blindness, may be the result of nutrient deficiencies in certain cases.

While exercise alone will not improve a severe condition, it may prevent a marginal vitamin or mineral deficiency from escalating into a larger problem which very well could prompt a condition such as cataracts.

The eyes, according to medical professionals, have one of the highest concentrations of nutrients of any organ of the body. It is essential, therefore, that one does everything possible to keep the supply of nourishment to the eye as constant and abundant as possible. Regular exercise does just that. It could be something as simple as walking for a little as 20 minutes several times a week.

Exercise is also a fantastic way to relieve stress— often the culprit in eye problems. Many people

241

experience stress-related cataracts (See page 157) If the doctor is perceptive and recognizes the formation as part of a reaction to a stressful situation, the formation will eventually subside once the person learns how to handle the problem which is troubling him.

Stress can also be the cause of one's eyes worsening when there is no organic reason for them to do so. Marc C., was an ambitious and highly motivated employee of a small computer firm in the Silicon Valley area of California. He was one of the top employees, in fact, of the company, with a highly visible and highly responsible position.

In the middle of a very important project, something went wrong with the storage of the data. Marc's computer had somehow lost every piece of vital information to this project, much of which was not duplicated anywhere else. It, indeed, was a stressful situation for this young man, as he spent days frantically trying to retrieve the lost data.

During this time, he noticed a distinct worsening of his vision. Already moderately myopic, this worried him. He visited a ophthalmologist who was alert enough to recognize the events occurring in Marc's life. The doctor told him, that in all probability, the decrease in vision was caused by the severe tension he was experiencing due to the lost data for the project. He advised Marc to postpone getting a new pair of glasses until the project had been completed.

After several months, the crisis passed. The data was re-assembled despite the computer foul up and the project completed only a few weeks behind the original schedule.

Marc's eyes soon improved. As he regained control of the project and the data were being re-collected, his eyesight gradually normalized to their previous state.

This, admittedly, is an extreme example of how tension can affect eyesight. In normal, more routine everyday circumstances one might not notice the changes in his vision. But, nonetheless, they probably are occurring.

Walking is one of the most effective tools in the treatment of stress. A recent study showed that corporate executives who took a 10 minute walk when feeling tensed received more benefits than those who just sat quietly or went for a cup of coffee or a candy bar. And the effects of the walk literally lasted for hours.

The Dr. Rinse Formula

It may seem odd to some that a food supplement

designed to strengthen ailing hearts also improves eyesight in some people. But it's true. The Dr. Rinse formula may help you better your visual acuity.

The formula, developed by Dr. Jacobus Rinse in response to his two heart attacks, works wonders on the entire human body. Listen to what Mrs. I.M.H. of Elizabeth, New Jersey, said about her eyesight, as well as the general condition of her health: "I was desperate and willing to try anything. I went on the Dr. Rinse Formula and within two weeks I noticed that I had increased stamina. Within a month, I was amazed to find myself reading something that I had not been able to read previously without my glasses. There was a general overall improvement in my condition . . ."

Mrs. G.V., of Cuthbert, Ga., experienced the same wonderful side effects using Dr. Rinse. "I was plagued with fatigue," she said, "poor circulation and arthritis. In addition, my eyesight continued to grow worse. After only several weeks of using the Dr. Rinse supplement, I discovered I was reading without my glasses. My arthritic pain is gone. Today I lead a far more active life than my children."

Grateful people have written Dr. Rinse thanking him because his supplement reversed their cataracts.

244

Dr. Rinse was a chemist, when at age 51, he was stricken with a heart attack. He didn't particularly like the idea of counting the years he had left. After all, the weekend of the attack, he was clearing the lot for his new house, so he read everything he could find on the subject of heart and heart attacks. He devised a formula, based upon his readings, but after several years suffered another heart attack.

Instead of giving in, Dr. Rinse read more and added necessary ingredients to his supplement. The result is that today literally thousands of people are alive and enjoying excellent eyesight in addition to robust health, thanks to Dr. Jacobus Rinse.

Testimonials from not only the United States, but from Europe, attest to the formula's success as a preventive.

The doctor receives letters of thanks for the results the formula have made, including reversing such conditions as high blood pressure, angina pectoris, diabetes, arthritis and obstructions in neck, leg and arm arteries. The end result of regular use of the doctor's formula appears to be the avoidance of heart attack, stroke and senility.

The Dr. Rinse Formula can be added to a variety of foods, such as yogurt, stews, soups, hot or cold cereals, cottage cheese, chunky applesauce,

245

scrambled eggs and even pancakes and waffles—either to the batter before cooking or sprinkle it on top of the cooked breakfast food.

Below is the recipe for the Dr. Rinse formula. The daily recommended dosage is a one-ounce serving. If you consider mixing your own too much trouble or time consuming, health food stores offer the original premixed Dr. Rinse Formula in 16 oz. cans — about a two-three week supply.

The Dr. Rinse Formula	
The Food Supplement	**The Quantity Per Day**
Lecithin	5 grams
Raw wheat germ	5 grams
Debittered brewer's yeast	5 grams
Bone meal	2 grams
Chopped sunflower seeds or oil	5 grams
Vitamin C	0.5 grams
Vitamin E	0.2 grams (200 IU)
Multi-vitamin-mineral tablet	one
Eventually to add anytime if extra nutrition desired:	
Bran flakes	5-10 grams
Kelp powder or tablets	1 gram
Zinc oxide	10 milligrams
Molasses, brown sugar, or honey as sweetening agent	6 grams (about 1 tablespoon) **2 Grams = 1 tablespoon**

Try this formula daily. For a synergistic effect, supplement it with a daily program of Aerobounding. The combination may just make you fell like a new person—and improve your vision.

Why Does The Dr. Rinse Formula Work?

It's easy to analyze the formula and discover why it is so beneficial to the body. Below is a quick note about the supplement's active ingredients.

Wheat Germ. Of all the cereals, wheat germ contributes the most to total, good health. It is rich in thiamin, riboflavin, niacin, protein, carbohydrates, fats and Vitamin E. One cup of raw wheat germ contains 25.5 grams of protein, more than is found in four ounces of turkey or two eggs or even a three-ounce steak. And combining this cereal with the other ingredients of the doctor's formula enriches its nutritional value.

Vitamin E. This vitamin has been known to reduce muscular pain and symptoms of fibrositis and may help prevent blood clots.

Vitamin C. Without this nutrient, capillaries would be fragile and display symptoms such as bleeding gums and bleeding under the skin. Vitamin C, moreover, lowers serum cholesterol, according to researchers and acts as a preventive in the formation of gallstones.

247

Bone Meal (ash). Because of its great natural calcium, bone meal is especailly good in the promotion of strong bones and teeth. It helps to regulate the heart beat and aids the skin. Other minerals found in bone meal include, zinc, cobalt, copper, sulphur, iodine, iron and manganese.

Brewer's Yeast. Rich in the B-Complex vitamins, such as pantothenic acid, Brewer's Yeast is also an excellent source of protein and several sulphur-containing amino acids. It also contains folic acid and inositol.

Lecithin. This substance also contains also the B-complex vitamins, choline and inositol. Lecithin is beneficial in reducing serum cholesterol. It may also be valuable in treating leg cramps and is a building block, essential for repairing weak cells and organs. This substance also helps the body to assimilate the Vitamins A and E.

Sunflower Seeds or Sunflower Oil. These are included for their rich content of unsaturated fats.

Garlic and the Eyes

Garlic has been a home remedy in many parts of Europe for centuries. Now scientists are also recognizing the value of this common plant and spice.

Modern research demonstrates that it is an excellent enhancer of circulation—many times a cause of common eye disorders—and helps to cleanse the blood.

Garlic, also, has been found to strengthen fragile blood vessels, such as those found in the eye, and help prevent recurring bleeding.

Physicians and nutritionists recommend a garlic clove or two daily or the addition of garlic capsules to their patients' daily vitamin regimen. One of the best is an old Bulgarian formula which combines pure garlic, hawthorn, rutin and hops. This natural formula contains only biologically-active garlic in an odorless form.

Flaxseed Oil

For additional insurance of healthy eyes, try cold-pressed unrefined flaxseed oil. It contains the essential fatty acids linoleic and linolenic acids, which have been associated with the improvement of many health problems, including those of the eye.

Unrefined, cold-pressed flaxseed oil may be

mixed with cottage cheese as a daily supplement.

This linseed oil is of high quality and offers the essential fatty acids the body needs. (But please do not heat, as this will destroy important elements in the oil.)

Kombucha

Another nutritional supplement which may help relieve eye problems is a natural fermented tea drink, currently one of the best selling natural health products in Europe. It's Kombucha. In addition to easing various eye problems, it also helps restore the entire system to good health.

It has already helped many Europeans overcome such diverse conditions as high cholesterol, impotence, prostate problems, migraine headaches, failing memory and lack of energy. For a more complete list of the many wonders Kombucha has been said to perform, see the box on page 234.

Kombucha works by strengthening the immune system and regulating one's metabolism. Among its active ingredients are glucoronic and lactic acids, as well as an array of most of the essential vitamins.

Glucoronic acid forms with substances in the

body—such as metabolic waste products and "poisonous" substances—to effectively eliminate them, producing a highly beneficial cleansing effect.

Moreover, the lactic acid helps maintain a healthy pH balance in the body. A deficiency of this acid may create health problems for the body. In Europe, lactic acid has been used as part of a comprehensive treatment for cancer. Dr. Veronica Carstens, M.D., the wife of the former West German president even "prescribes" Kombucha for her cancer patients, citing that "the lactic acid in the natural tea drink is very important to my patients' treatments."

Recent studies link low levels of lactic acid and alkaline blood readings with heightened susceptibility to tumor formation.

The recommended daily dosage of Kombucha is three glasses daily—one with breakfast and the other two glasses prior to the afternoon and evening meals.

Sylvia Rottenau had suffered from severe depression for many years. Her doctor suggested she take Kombucha for her unrelated stomach and gallbladder problems. Not only did her stomach and gallbladder improve, but "after only a few weeks on Kombucha, my depression completely disappeared," she said.

Sylvia reports that not only did she use the natural tea drink faithfully, but she has her two sons drink it also. Their academic performance improved dramatically after just several weeks and most surprisingly to Sylvia, was that her children were able to see much better.

Kombucha is the result of a natural process of the fermentation of a specific plant, just as wine the result of the fermentation of grapes.

Dr. Reinhold Wiesner, M.D., used the beverage on 264 of his seriously ill patients who did not respond to other medications. These people suffered from a variety of ailments, including gout, rheumatism, impotency, arteriosclerosis, cancer and infectious diseases. Kombucha helped everyone of the doctor's patients. "What Kombucha did for my patients," he said, "no hospital can accomplish."

Kombucha was "discovered" by Dr. Rudolf Sklenar of Germany, who as a young army officer in World War II, was stationed in several Eastern European countries, including parts of Russia. Sklenar was impressed with the good health of the peasants in these areas, especially in contrast to his fellow Germans who had lived their lives in cities. Indeed, it was not at all unusual for the peasants to live healthy, productive lives of 90, even 100 years or more. They were not crippled by arthritis or debilitated with bad hearts as was common in many cities in Western Europe. Even the incidence of the common cold and the flu was extremely low.

During his stay in these countries, Dr. Sklenar observed that the peasants drank a fruity drink with every meal. He asked and was told it was Kombucha. The natives credited this drink with providing them with long, healthy lives.

Obviously skeptical at first, Sklenar, nonetheless, learned to cultivate the plant from which it was made and to ferment the drink. He returned to Germany at the end of the war with his new-found product and began administering it to patients on whom all other medications had failed. Much to his pleasure, Kombucha really did work. It relieved many chronic conditions and helped his patients return to good health, something some of them has not known in years.

It was not long before word spread throughout Germany of the young doctor's "miracle cures." He was treating people not only from all parts of the nation, but from every corner of the earth.

And since its release commercially on the European market in 1987, it has become one of the best-selling natural health products of all time.

Kombucha is finally available in the United States. For more information on this amazing all-natural drink, check with your local health food store or health food catalog. They should be able to direct you to a good reliable source.

The Amazing Natural Remedies of Kombucha

Listed below are the conditions Kombucha has been able to help for thousands of people across the European continent. This naturally-fermented tea drink is free of any adverse side effects and one may be able to see results after a remarkable short period of time.

Arthritis • Arteriosclerosis • Multiple Sclerosis •Migraine Headaches • Kidney Problems • Gout • Acne • Eczema • Digestive Problems • Hypertension • Obesity • Menstrual Problems • Eye Problems • Failing Memory • Fatigue • Liver and Gallbladder Ailments • Rheumatism • Bladder Problems • Varicose Veins • Impotence • Prostate Inflammation • High Cholesterol and much more.

Herbs/Vitamins

Another nutritional supplement which may help to create healthy eyes is Herbs/Vitamins. Like Kombucha, it's a European creation, developed by Dr. Fleming Norgaard, M.D., D.D.S.

Dr. Norgaard's credentials are impeccable. He was the first person in his homeland of Denmark to earn two doctorates of science degrees—one in medicine the other in odontology, the science which deals with the structure, health and growth of teeth. In fact, his original research and ideas in odontology laid the foundation for the current treatment of patients who have problems in their temples.

Dr. Norgaard developed Herb/Vitamin over a period of several decades, testing it on himself first and later his wife and friends, before subjecting the supplement to the rigorous standards of the medical community.

Herb/Vitamin's capabilities include boosting the immune system—which makes one more resistant to colds and infections, relieves the symptoms of asthma and hay fever, helps reduce pain due to arthritis and strengthens nails, hair and skin. These are just a few of its many abilities.

A precise blend of herbs and vitamins, this "multi-potent" supplement works from the inside out, restoring ailing cells and tissues. Its effects are noticed quickly—restored energy, better skin, less aches and pains.

Just three tablets daily may not only increase one's vitality and improve the circulatory system, but it may also help build healthier eyes.

Esther P., took Herb/Vitamin because she was experiencing inexplicable hair loss. After two weeks, her hair not only was growing back healthier than ever, but her eyesight had improved. "I was able to read very fine print which before has eluded me," she exclaimed enthusiastically.

An added benefit of using Herb/Vitamin daily is its ability to slow the aging process. Dr. Norgaard likes to recall the story of an elderly gentleman who has been an invalid for several years. For two years this man had literally been condemned to lead a life from his bed, unable to get up for any reason.

"After only two short weeks on my tablets," the doctor explained, "the man was able to stand up and, indeed, was quite mobile. Within a very short period of time, in fact, he resumed his former social life as if there had been no interruption. To look at him today, you would not be able to tell he had ever been ill, much less confined to bed."

Stress, we noted elsewhere in this book, is, indeed a danger to eyesight. Exercise can help ward off the evil consequences of tension, but to add extra insurance, one may also consider taking the Herb/Vitamin "multi-potent" supplement.

"Using my supplement," Dr. Norgaard noted, "can reduce those negative influences caused by the pressures of today's hectic lifestyle." If you are under much stress and feel a little rundown, the doctor suggests doubling the dosage of Herb/ Vitamin for a few days. "You will soon be back to normal," he said.

In fact, with regular use of this supplement, one may very well prevent the negative side effects of stress, such as poor eyesight and temporary impairment of one's mental abilities, the doctor commented.

Other Conditions Improved

The following is a quick summary of some of the many ailments Herb/Vitamin has eased for Europeans.

1) *Degenerative Arthritis*

Some people experience "rapid, distinct improvement in their conditions," according to Dr. Norgaard. The increased energy, and vitality the tablets provide prompt the arthritis victim to increase his physical

257

activities. Movement is one of the best therapies for joints struck by the painful disease.

2) *Inflammation of the Prostate Gland*

Most men beyond the age of 50 suffer from this uncomfortable and dangerous condition. Accompanying the inflammation is painful urination or the inability to urinate, the latter a very real health danger. Dr. Norgaard's formula may help ease the problem due to its effective action upon the bladder muscles.

3) *Incontinence*

Many older women—and some younger ones, as well—suffer from this embarassing problem. The regular use of Herbs/Vitamins, Dr. Norgaard said, may, indeed, free these women from this condition.

4) *Urinary Tract Infections*

Herb/Vitamin may be able to relieve the symptoms of this infection. It allows for the elimination of the urine and its disease-producing bacteria. It works equally well on men as women, the doctor said.

5) *Female Complaints*

Both pre-menstrual pains and the problems associated with menopause may be eased with regular use of this "multi-potent" tablet. Because the pill is made of nothing but natural ingredients, it is a vastly better alternative than the use of potentially-dangerous hormones. Dr. Norgaard notes that Herbs/Vitamins has provided relief even when hormones would not help some women.

6) *Heart and Circulatory Problems*

> A high degree of improvement has been accomplished in many people, following regular use of Herb/Vitamins, the Dane noted. It allows for a better flow of blood to the heart because of the dilating effect on the heart muscles by the tablets' ingredients.

If you are interested in learning more about this Herb/Vitamin, check with your local health food store or health food catalog. They should be able to direct you to a good reliable source for these wonderful new Herb/Vitamin combination tablets from Denmark.

Lighting and Your Body

The artifical light that most of us are exposed to on a regular basis has effects that reach farther than just causing tired eyes.

Tests and studies conclude that cool fluorescent lighting—popular in most offices and public areas—may cause a host of health problems, including cavaties!

While on the surface that may not seem possible—consider, for a moment, the effects of natural sunlight upon the body. Light stimulates the pituitary and pineal glands and, researchers say, perhaps even other areas of the mid-brain which control the production of other hormones.

259

The pineal gland is a little known organ, located deep within the brain. It secretes the hormone called melatonin, which is responsible for signalling the onset of puberty and also serves as the body's internal timekeeper. Melatonin also induces sleep and influences moods.

It has just been learned within the last decade that bright, natural light slows down the production of melatonin while darkness increases it.

When the retina is stimulated by visible light, some of the nerve impulses produced travel along the optic nerve to the visual area of the brain which then interprets what we see.

Other impulses, however, travel from the optic nerve to the hypothalamus, which controls the body's internal environment including the pituitary gland. And this gland, in turn, regulates the endocrine system.

This process occurs not only with the aid of the portion of the visible spectrum, but also by the bands of light which we can't detect with the naked eye. It's what we don't see—and what we aren't receiving with conventional fluorescent lights— that are causing problems.

Look, for a moment, at the more obvious benefits of sunlight. Studies in the last decade have confirmed that sunlight plays a major role in the body's absorption of calcium, and the maintenance of our biological rhythms and even our emotional stability. Those afflicted with Seasonal Affective Disorder—more commonly called SAD—are treated with "artificial sunlight" or full spectrum fluorescent light.

In a study of elderly veterans, researchers at Massachusetts General Hospital in Boston discovered the effect of artificial lighting upon calcium absorption. For calcium to be of any use to the body, Vitamin D3 must also be present.

Also called Cholecalciferol, Vitamin D3 isn't a vitamin at all. It's a hormone whose production is stimulated by sunlight, specifically, by the ultraviolet rays in sunlight.

Headed by Robert Neer, the doctors divided the men into two groups. One was exposed to artificial sunlight—which included the ultraviolet rays—and the other to ordinary indoor lighting.

Those receiving the artificial sunlight had a 15 percent *increase* in calcium absorption compared to the 25 percent *decrease* experienced by the group exposed to the indoor lighting.

Tips For Lighting A Room

We've all experienced the sensation of tired eyes, whether because we stayed up too long watching that late-late movie or we spent too many hours involved in intensive reading. The following are several tips to help prevent those tired eyes and to help you receive the maximum effect from the lighting in your home or office:

1) Overhead lighting, which illuminates the entire room or work space, is the number one criteria to ensure ease while reading.

2) The amount of illumination needed depends upon the color of the walls in the room. The darker the color, the more light that is required. An average-sized room for example, with light-toned walls, requires approximately 150 to 200 watts of overhead lighting. A handy rule of thumb is to remember that no part of the room should be in darkness.

3) Overhead lighting may be supplemented with floor or desk lamps. Be sure, though, that the bulbs are shaded so the eye is not directly exposed to the light.

4) When writing or reading, use a standing lamp, placed about two feet behind what you are working on, and about a foot to the left of your shoulders. Experts agree that 150-watt is optimum. If you use a desk or gooseneck lamp,

---

Tips For Lighting A Room (Con't)

---

it needs to be only half that wattage—about 75—and should be set about a foot above the reading material.

5) Avoid, whenever possible, using white paper on a dark desk. Instead, use a blotter of medium tone to reduce the amount of contrast.

The Liver Responds to Light

The liver responds to environmental light in several ways. The organ's ability to detoxify harmful drugs is different under certain lights. More laboratory rats die of poisoning when kept in darkened rooms or exposed to abnormal light-dark cycles than when housed in bright light.

Of those rats in bright light that do die, fewer deaths occur after they have received eight hours of light.

In humans, the use of full-spectrum lighting helps infants recover from neonatal jaundice. In the 1950s a nurse in England noticed that when newborns were taken outside, their jaundice quickly disappeared. At about the same time, another professional discovered that sunlight could bleach

263

out—and destroy—bilirubin in test tubes. When the liver malfunctions, bilirubin, a yellowish pigment is produced upon the death of red blood cells. This pigment builds up in the tissues, and is responsible for the yellow tint associated with jaundice.

It was not until the late 1960s, however, that peditrician Jerold Lucey of the University of Vermont in Burlington confirmed those findings. Babies exposed to full spectrum lighting for several days actually experience a decrease in bilirubin levels.

This type of treatment—using full spectrum lighting to help the body achieve health—is called *phototherapy.*

It's been around since the ancient Greeks, but did not gain the approval of the scientific community until the early 20th century. In 1903, Neils Finsen of Denmark won the Nobel Prize for the use of light to cure disease. The doctor had observed that tubercular skin lesions were common in the winter in Norway, but not in the summer. He developed "Finsen Light" which closely simulated natural sunlight. The invention was highly effective.

In the 1940s, however, the use of light as a bacteria killing agent was all but abandoned, because of the advent of antibiotics—at least in this country. Countries subjected to extended periods of darkness—such as Scandanavia and parts of Russia—still use phototherapy. In fact, many residents of these countries routinely complain of "sunlight starvation." This condition is characterized by a general weakening of the body's muscles, the presence of frequent minor illnesses, fatigue, and chronic irritiblity.

The Russians and Germans are so convinced of natural light's health benefits, in fact, that underground miners are mandated by law to take phototherapy as an aid in battling black lung disease.

Living with Artificial Light

These findings might lead one to ask what the effects are of living practically entirely in artificial light—as many of us do.

Indoor lighting is vastly different from sunlight, as we have seen. It is not as bright. A typical office might be lit with 600 to 700 lux (the international unit that measures illumination). Moreover, artificial light lacks the entire range of the spectrum. Fluorescent lights have very little ultraviolet rays. They also, many times, produce an irritating bluish or greenish cast to the room. Incadescent bulbs— the standard light bulb with which most homes are lit—receive the majority of their energy in the infrared part of the spectrum.

Unfortunately, little is known about the long-term effects of prolonged exposure to artificial light.

Dr. Richard Wurtman, of the Massachusetts Institute of Technology, suggests that more information be found. Dr. Wurtman is an endocrinologist, renowned for his work on biological rhythms, the pineal gland and the biological effects of light.

"Only miniscule sums have been expended to characterize and exploit the biological effects of light," he has asserted. "Very little has been done to protect citizens against potentially harmful or biologically inadequate lighting environments."

He believes that in several generations, we will be feeling the effects of "light pollution." Recent studies, in fact, seem to bear out his premise. Fluorescent lighting has been associated with higher levels of hormones responsible for stress, eye problem and hyperactivity in children.

Some nutritionists speculate, moreover, that cool fluorescent lighting uses up large quantities of Vitamin A, which can eventually lead to night blindness.

Some nutritionists have even linked the decreased Vitamin A supply caused by sustained fluorescent light exposure to skin blemishes.

Criteria for Evaluation

Four criteria are to be considered when determining artificial light's impact upon humans:

1) Intensity of the light

2) Wave lengths of light

3) Time of Exposure

4) Duration of Exposure

Obviously, the more time people spend in artificial light, the greater the possible effects. One of the places that children spend a large part of their time is at school. Recently, studies have been conducted using *Vita-Lite* full spectrum lights and ordinary, cool fluroscent light.

Vita-Lite closely simulates natural sunlight, providing the full range of wavelengths both visible and invisible in a proportion that is the most similar to sunlight.

An elementary school in Sarasota, Florida, used four classrooms to discover the effects of full spectrum lighting.

Vita-Lite was used in two of the classrooms, while the other two retained the conventional cool white fluorescent lights.

After a very short time, the effects were extremely noticeable. In the classroom with the conventional lighting, the students experienced nervous fatigue, irritability, a great deal of hyper-activity and short attention spans.

By contrast, the students who worked under the full spectrum lights had markedly improved behavior patterns, as well as higher academic performances. And, perhaps most surprising of all, fewer cavaties than the other group of students.

A separate study conducted in a British Columbia school system produced similar results. In this case, however, the Wetaskiwin School District used four different elementary schools and tested a variety of combinations of environmental conditions, including the use of *Vita-Lite*.

Students were tested prior to the study and then behavior, academic performance and vision were closely monitored for 10 months.

There were significant improvements in the students whose school used the *Vita-Lite* full spectrum lighting. Noise levels were significantly lower, with the children being more well behaved.

Those who worked under the *Vita-Lite* also had demonstrably more positive moods than those who attended other schools. Moreover, there was a lower absenteeism rate among certain grade levels in the buildings with the full spectrum lighting.

And, as in the school in Florida, the students had fewer cavities than other children who worked under regular indoor lighting. Scientists have not yet determined why full spectrum lighting would inhibit the formation of cavities.

Eye Health Natural Prevention And Treatment Guide	
Vitamins and Minerals	*How They Work:*
Vitamin A	Prevents night blind ness and problems with the cornea.
Vitamin B-Complex	May help alleviate amblyopia, chronic watery eyes, blood shot eyes and decrease sensitivity to light.
Vitamin D/Calcium	Used in conjunction to treat nearsightedness.
Herbal Remedies	
Herb	*Use:*
Yarrow Tea	May help watery eyes, may relieve pain behind the eyes.

Herbal Remedies (Con't)	
Chamomile Compress	May reduce eye pain and remove bags under the eyes.
Mallow Compress	May help relieve strained tired eyes.
Calamus Juice	May strengthen eyes.
Other Natural Methods	*How They Work*
Unrefined, Cold-Pressed Flaxseed Oil	Great source of essential fatty acids—linoleic and linolenic—needed for overall good health.
Garlic	Strengthens fragile blood vessels of the eye.
Dr. Rinse Formula	Has been known to help circulatory problems as well as improve eyesight.
Kombucha	Strengthens immune system. Has been known to help various eye problems.
Herbs/Vitamins	Natural Supplement, may help circulation problems, sometimes a cause of eye problems.

Other Natural Methods (Con't)

Exercise

Any exercise is good because it improves poor circulation, sometimes a cause of eye problems.

Chapter 11

Dr. Salov's Visionary Therapies

The natural modern opthamologist must use the eyes as the opening or mirror into the health of the whole person.

Just as this edition of *Hidden Secrets For Better Vision* was nearing completion, I met a Wisconsin ophthalmologist whose years of successful, alternative visual therapies have restored eyesight to hundreds of patients, while bringing him international recognition.

I believe the simple, straightforward methods used by Dr. Leslie H. Salov merit coverage in a book of this scope. They enlighten concepts covered in previous chapters, and can easily be implemented by those already using Bates exercises, vitamin and nutritional therapies.

Leslie H. Salov, MD, is an unassuming character - the kind of fellow you might meet in a coffee shop over newspapers and breakfast. He's the

272

man with well-set opinions, thought-out responses to every question, and a wry wit to make even hard-to-understand concepts go down easily.

But Dr. Salov is no lightweight. He has conducted eye problem studies at clinics and universities throughout Europe and the United States. His resume includes stints as staff physician at the New Jersey State Mental Hospital; primary researcher in diabetic retinopathy at Montefiore Hospital, Pittsburgh; ophthamological consultant for the Atomic Energy Commission; and lecturer to Walter Reed Army Medical Center and London University College Hospital Medical School. Dr. Salov has published dozens of papers in medical journals, and has written five medical textbooks. His expertise extends beyond ophthalmology, and he has successfully treated patients whose eye problems were simply symptoms of other physical problems.

What makes this ophthalmologist different from the rest is his approach to eye medicine. Dr. Salov treats the entire body - not just the relatively small proportion that is causing visual problems. Dr. Salov's approach to ophthalmology is deeply influenced by his friend and instructor Dr. Hans Goldmann, a world renowned professor of ophthalmology at the medical school of Berne, Switzerland. Just as nutritional advocates preach, Dr. Salov practices building up the immune system, flushing out built-up toxins and revitalizing the repair and maintenance mechanisms every healthy body starts out with.

But Dr. Salov adds on therapies practiced in Eastern and Western Europe, India, and China, as well as North American approaches to stress management and autonomic nerve reflex response.

Dr. Salov left his standard medical practice in the mid-1970's, but he did not retire - he opened two Vision Centers on opposite ends of the nation! Dr. Salov continues to shuttle between Wisconsin and Florida, treating patients using an intensive, one-on-one program, conducting research, and meeting with television and newspaper reporters to spread the news on how to maintain sharp vision throughout a long life by treating the "whole person," body, mind, and spirit.

Here are a few examples of the work Dr. Salov is doing today; as written by Dr. Salov himself.

THE LAWYER'S CATARACTS

Robert Brown, a Boston attorney in his late 70's, came to see me at my center in Whitewater, Wisconsin, in the late 1980's. He had cataracts and was frightened of surgery, he said, having seen what happens when an operation doesn't work out as planned.

"My brother was operated on for cataracts about a year ago, and went completely blind after the operation. He had two detachments of his retinas," he told me. "I'm not saying it's the doctor's fault, but he never saw again. I don't want to go through that. I'm scared to death," Brown added.

"I only want one thing when this is all over," he said. "I live four blocks from my office. I want to be able to safely drive my car from my house to my office. I want to feel that I'm still part of the world, and driving is an important part of that. Can you help me?"

"You are going to help yourself," I told him.

I listed all the methods Brown would learn during his stay at our vision center in Whitewater. Human - Bio - Feed - Back or Visualization therapy teaches the autonomic nervous system to increase blood flow to the ophthalmic arteries. Improved nutrition, using natural, organic vegetarian foods, heavy on fresh juices, to cleanse the body and build up the immune system. Deep abdominal breathing, stress control and relaxation techniques complete the therapy.

"I am going to ask you to do all these difficult things," I told Mr. Brown. "If you do these things, you will be privileged to have improvement. If you don't do these things, you won't."

The choice was simple enough for Mr. Brown. After a week at our Center, Brown returned to his

275

practice in Boston. He stayed on the strict vegetarian diet and continued the meditative relaxation therapy. Six months later he called me.

"I want you to know that today, I drove my car from my home to my office," he said. "I want to thank you. You did the only thing there was to do for me."

That's all there was to the conversation. I hear from him now and then, by notes he sends. Once in a while he writes to say he's still driving to his office every morning. He's now in his mid-80's, and is still very active in his work.

Glaucoma Patient Saved from Blindness
Miss Carlucci's Glaucoma

Elizabeth Carlucci was a 34-year old New Jersey school teacher, mother of a delightful 6 year old daughter. The pair lived with Carlucci's parents in suburban Elizabeth, New Jersey. Miss Carlucci had a problem.

Elizabeth's doctor found that extremely high pressure was robbing her of her eyesight - a severe form of glaucoma that does not respond well to surgery or drugs. This young woman faced complete blindness within two years - and her vision was already deteriorated so severely she feared walking around the block with her little girl.

Her increasing handicap cost her job. She became depressed, and eventually housebound. The best ophthalmologists in New York and New Jersey confirmed her doctor's diagnosis. Finally, Elizabeth's parents implored me to keep their daughter from going completely blind.

After careful examination and thought, I decided to use a very strict plan of therapy which has been used in different parts of the world for a number of years. This treatment is usually reserved for cancer patients. It is a fasting procedure, (When one eats nothing and only drinks water for this period) which necessitated her parents' full cooperation and my constant supervision. Elizabeth agreed to consume nothing but water for several days, remain very quiet and maintain a loving, happy environment for the duration.

Miss Carlucci fasted for 24 days. I monitored her condition daily, measuring eye pressure, circulation, optic nerve condition and her general constitution. (The reader is warned never to begin a fast without medical supervision.)

After the fifteenth day of fasting, the pressure in Elizabeth's eyes began to reduce. On day 20, it reached normal. It remained normal until the end of the fast. Over several weeks, fresh, organic fruits, juices and eventually vegetables were added to her diet. She remains a vegetarian to this day, and has converted her parents and daughter to the practice, as well.

Best of all, Elizabeth Carlucci's glaucoma is gone, and her vision remains clear. Despite the orthodox doctors' gloomy, hopeless prognoses, this woman's willingness and cooperation with an alternative therapy saved her eyesight - and her career.

Tumor in the Brain Affected Eyesight — Healed Without Surgery
A Secretary's Victory

Secretary Janis Wells 42, also regained her vision using methods learned at our vision center in Wisconsin.

Wells had a long history of good health, so she was surprised when, periodically through the spring of 1992, her left hand grew warm and tingly. She started having trouble seeing movement to her left, and her vision became blurry on that side.

After consulting with two specialists and undergoing several tests, a brain scan revealed a tumor just above her pituitary gland, in her brain. This is where the optic nerves cross one another - an area imperative to vision.

Surgery proved difficult. Doctors told Janis they could not remove the tumor without damaging her vision and glandular functions. But, thankfully, a biopsy of the tumor tissue revealed no cancer tissue. The growth was a "neuro-glioma," a non-malignant tumor that could, through continued growth, cost her vision and endocrine health, and cause paralysis of the extremities. The doctors bombarded the tumor with radiation and chemotherapy, but to little effect. Months later, they sent her home, saying they could not stop the tumor or save her vision. (The orthodox doctors reported that the tumor had doubled in size after Janis had been treated with radiation and chemotherapy.) It was then that Janis reported to our Vision and Health Center. At that point, the tumor in her head measured 3/4 of an inch in diameter.

Janis was given no medications or surgery. She started onto a natural vegetarian diet, and studied methods of human-bio-feed-back that enabled her to send her body's specialized healing cells directly to the tumor. She learned breathing techniques that helped her to relax and expel stress and waste from her system. Her spirits were bolstered by family therapy, which increased the harmony in her home and helped her to remain on our program of modern, natural, alternative therapies.

Over several months of outpatient therapy, Janis continued to have Magnetic Resonance Imaging (MRI) scans performed on the glioma area. (As she had done before she saw me). Very gradually, the tumor decreased its size. After four months of my alternative therapy, the tumor disappeared from the scan. Images taken every six months since then reveal no reoccurrence. Janis' eyesight and glandular functions are now normal. Several years after this alternative treatment, the brain scan showed that the tumor had been completely absorbed.

Medical Doctor's Eyesight Completely Restored with Dr. Salov's Therapy

The Ophthalmologist's Ophthalmologist

Finally comes the testimonial report of Jim Okunberg, M.D., an ophthalmologist from Louisiana.

Jim, a medical school graduate, was in his first year of specialized study to become an ophthalmologist when he started having difficulty seeing during delicate eye surgery procedures. He had his instructor examine his eyes. The news wasn't good - the young doctor had keratoconus: bulging, misshapen corneas that result in extreme vision loss.

Surrounded by the finest eye practitioners, Jim had them design special corrective contact lenses to treat his problem. After six months of itchy, watering eyes, Jim realized his vision wasn't improving, and that the contact lenses were totally useless. His teachers at the University had no other advice or suggestions for treatment.

Jim said he had second thoughts about our treatments, but no other options. He spent two weeks at our Florida center, consuming high quality, fresh vegetarian meals, soothing his medical school stresses, mastering the human-bio-feed-back, "guided imagery" techniques that send healing leukocytes (important immune cells of his own body) to the damaged eye tissues.

The young doctor's mastery of eye anatomy helped him visualize the needed repairs. Jim could, through the mental imagery, improve his eye tissues' uptake of needed nutrition from his blood supply. And thus the patient was first to notice when the hyaline bands, which hold the cornea in its normal position in his cornea, began returning to their normal function. He gradually overcame the malformed cone formations as well, and saw his vision restored to normal.

All this took five months. After finishing the treatment, Dr. Jim Okunberg continued his studies, graduated and established a thriving ophthalmology practice. Ten years later, he reports no recurrence of symptoms or decrease in clear vision.

In a written thank-you testimonial, Okunberg told me, "I shall be everlastingly grateful to you and the program for the good results I received."

My files contain similar letters from former patients who've regained at least partial vision after diagnoses of macular degeneration, diabetic retinopathy, cataracts, retinitis pigmentosa and iritis. After successfully treating patients as varied as old-time Hollywood starlet Gloria Swanson, Pittsburgh steelworkers whose eyes were injured in industrial accidents, a dentist whose corneas were burned by acid and children born blind as a result of cerebral palsy, I consider them a testimony to my methods.

I developed this combination, alternative program of therapy during the 1970's, after developing macular degeneration. My fellow doctors told me that my case was untreatable.

I looked over research done with Professor Hans Goldmann, at the medical school in Bern, Switzerland, and tried several therapies he used in the past with patients like Carlucci and Okunberg.

My vision is not perfect, but at 95% percent acuity it's not bad for someone who developed macular degeneration. There is no condition that cannot be improved upon, in varying degrees, given the proper therapy, education and personal commitment to following the program.

Chapter 12

Dr. Salov's Secrets

The whole is greater than the sum of its parts, and the eyes are only part of the whole person. In order to improve vision, it is essential to improve the health of the whole person simultaneously.

How does one convey an understanding of Mankind's body, mind and spirit? It's a difficult task to sum up Dr. Salov's methods, as they employ concepts that seem foreign to us clinical, cynical Westerners. We are accustomed to doctors treating our symptoms, not investigating the causes of our diseases and complaints, and especially not our emotions, attitudes and spiritual selves.

But alternative treatments like Dr. Salov's work on principals that reach back to ancient Greece, and extend through physicians and philosophers like Hippocrates, Galen, Katzentackus and Paracelsus.

Even these ancients knew the body is a set of interlocking systems that produce their own

283

protective substances. Paracelsus, for instance, understood that tears protect the eyes from invading illness. Modern science tells us that tears comprise more than 30 different chemicals, including lysosomes, natural ocular antibiotics. This natural physician of the 17th century also knew that our immune system carries certain specialized cells which act as very important antibiotics in healing and curing diseases of the human being.

We know that leukocytes - white blood cells produced in bone marrow - produce an enzyme called dismutase, the most powerful natural antibiotic in the world. The body also creates "universal cells," called fibroblasts." Paracelsus, physician to royal families in Austria and Hungary, knew about fibroblasts, even though he never called them by that name. Today, Dr. Salov helps patients make use of their fibroblasts as part of a modern, natural therapy for serious diseases like macular degeneration, glaucoma, and diabetic retinopathy.

Our own century has seen great developments in the healing powers of spirituality and philosophy as well as the sciences of physiology, chemistry and biology. The qualities of natural foods, environment, interpersonal relationships and personal spirituality have proven effects on human health. The need for "inner peace" to maintain health has gained importance as doctors realize the healthy body needs to balance physical, emotional and spiritual elements. Use of natural approaches to "the whole person" has gained respect among the most clinical of modern doctors, as practitioners of techniques like human-bio-feed-back, visualization and natural nutrition show themselves effective.

How does this effect the eyes? One good example is glaucoma, a condition that can cause complete blindness because of high ocular pressure in the eye caused by a build up of fluid that cannot drain properly. Most eye doctors would recommend surgery to relieve the high ocular pressure in the eye, but a natural, alternative practitioner will look at the patient's lifestyle and use modern, natural therapies to gradually lower the pressure and restore normal vision. Dr. Salov says most glaucoma patients are intelligent professionals who lead stressful, busy lives. They take little notice of their diets or general health until their vision begins to weaken.

The patient who consults Dr. Salov or other alternative ophthalmologists finds them examining every aspect of his life - not just his eyes. He'll be taught to relax, using taped messages, special color therapies and music. He'll discuss his relationships with spouse, family and co-workers, and learn how to peacefully co-exist with them. He'll learn anatomy, digestion and nutrition, and will see his dinner plate heaped with garden produce rather than fatty meat. He'll be taught a special deep breathing technique, and will take regular exercise as part of his "eye treatment." He'll gather with other patients to master meditation as well as the self-healing technique called human-bio-feed-back or visualization.

"We've followed these methods over the past 30 years, and we're very convinced that if the patients follow the natural, intelligent therapy we advise, usually the glaucoma is improved and the pressure in the eye returns to normal," Dr. Salov said. "The aqueous fluid can then be properly drained from the eye and the patient's vision returns to normal."

Orthodox medicine treats glaucoma as an entity rather than a symptom, Dr. Salov said. Eye drops and surgeries attempt to lower pressure in the eye, but these treatments simply create a chronic condition, often leading to blindness.

STEP BY STEP with Dr. Salov

I believe the only way to heal all types of eye disease is through concentrated, one-on-one therapy - like that provided at inpatient clinics. A week at one of our centers includes all or most of the procedures outlined below.

COMMUNICATION

After initial physical exams and paperwork are completed, I simply talk with my patients - discussing relationships, workplace, hobbies and emotions. I take careful notes on just what creates stress reactions in the patient, as stress and depression are known to deplete immune system integrity.

Attitudes, lighting conditions, living and work environments are also considered for their possible effects on visual health. These specifics are used when making audio tapes designed to relax the patient and guide him through healing therapies tailored to his individual needs. When the patient goes home, he can work to correct all the elements that add to his problem. Everything from poor lighting to family feuds.

NEW DIETARY PROCEDURES

The patient's physical condition is considered carefully before an individual dietary plan is formed. I recommend drinking daily servings of fresh, organic fruit and vegetable juices. Recipes and preparation instructions help our patients to continue in this regimen when their treatment at our Vision & Health Center is finished and they return home.

We insist on a meat-free diet since various studies have found that chemical dyes, growth hormones and antibiotics in supermarket meat are very harmful. We also tell our patients to purchase only naturally grown, organic, fresh produce, as processed and canned produce are often subject to sprays of pesticides, herbicides, preservatives and sometimes even radioactive rays.

Our regimen of "super nutrition" is meant to make the immune system stronger and increase the production of our bodies' natural healing elements.

Anatomy Lessons

We conduct a careful tutorial, showing in detail just how our eyes function in relation to the rest of the body. The patient's own condition is examined and explained, using graphics, diagrams and charts. The processes that damaged the patient's eyes are shown clearly, as well as the anatomical changes that must take place to restore vision.

Biofeedback and Visualization

Careful anatomy teaching is put to good use when human-bio-feed-back begins. Through this meditative exercise, the patient uses his mind to direct his body to heal itself. It works for most who use it with dedication and consistency!

A human being with his mind can actually relax the little muscles in the walls of his Canal of Schlemm and excrete the extra fluid inside his eye so glaucoma pressure is relieved. That's why ophthalmologists use eye drops - when the pupil of the eye is small, the filter inside the eye opens up and sends the extra fluid into the Canal of Schlemm.

But you know what happens chronically after years of using those drops? Pieces of the iris break off and go inside the eye. They produce infections, create blockage, and prevent the aqueous fluid from leaving the eye. So, you see, the essence of the treatment used by orthodox physicians is, in itself, a horrible catastrophe. It's not understood that the human being can be taught to relax, to keep his pupils small, to open up the Canal of Schlemm and bring the fluid out without any chemical help or surgery thus reducing the damagingly high ocular pressure in the eye.

Several years ago, I treated a year-old Cherokee Indian boy named Paco, who was born with a cataract in one eye. His mother agreed to follow my prescriptions faithfully. Five months after starting the therapy, the baby's eye was normal. The little boy's developing language skills latched onto visualization concepts naturally.

You can't teach a little baby biofeedback, you

can't teach him visualization. But you can get the message to him by making a tape, which I did. The baby listened to it constantly - a story about the whole body contributing to building up an immune system, getting the bone marrow rich with leukocytes, and getting those leukocytes to the eye, where they could heal.

We teach our patient's about their own important immune cells such as leukocytes. Leukocytes are tiny, moveable cells that produce a powerful enzyme - dismutase - that can destroy the outer coverings of viruses and bacteria and kill them. A leukocyte can change its shape and surround and engulf bacteria, viruses and infections. Thousands and thousands of them can attack tumors, absorb blood, destroy tumor cells and absorb the waste and take it away to be expelled, through our breath, our skin pores, through our urine and feces. These are marvelous, powerful mechanisms that the orthodox physician and the ophthalmologist either don't know or don't appreciate. Our leukocytes can also destroy, dissolve and absorb cataracts, as they did in the case of Paco.

Adults also use tapes. The patient daily settles into a quiet state and summons a mental image of the damaged areas in his eye, then mentally directs blood, oxygen and those miraculous leukocytes to the very part that most needs repair. This "guided imagery" system is used to stimulate the body's immunity to attack impurities and repair damaged tissue.

Human-bio-feed-back, guided imagery and visualization have common roots. They all draw on the concept of using the conscious mind to control the autonomic (involuntary) processes that usually occur automatically inside our bodies. They are not common practices in medical clinics throughout the world. But special places such as the Menninger Clinic of Topeka, Kansas, and our Vision and Health Centers, teach these important therapies.

MEDITATION

Meditation is another practice fundamental to our therapy.

Meditation is the conscious throwing-off of the day's worries and stresses, the emptying of the mind of concerns and consciousness. It creates a deep state of relaxation and feelings of peace and well-being.

Unbeknown to us, daily stresses create repeated automatic chemical changes in our bodies. Arteries contract and decrease blood and oxygen flow. Metabolism suffers. The eye, always super sensitive to changes in oxygen levels, may over time develop "floaters," tiny breaks in the eye's blood vessels that appear as small, black dots of different shapes which create greater visual problems, as well as a host of other complaints.

I believe that meditation is necessary for every individual who has special eye and health problems. It is important for people with such problems to meditate daily. Meditation cleanses you from all the "gloom" that's been around you from the negative people, pollution and anxiety of living. This "gloom" clogs the neural "highway" that carries information to and from the brain. A session of meditation and visualization can clear the road, creating an improved pathway for ideas and nerve impulses to travel with ease over all the nerves.

I recommend certain "props" to help meditation work. Wear comfortable, loose clothing. Find a cool spot, away from bright light and drafts. Unplug the telephone. Send the kids to a movie. But don't get too comfortable, or you'll fall asleep!

Use a straight-backed chair with arms, and equip your "space" with pleasant items; a vase of flowers, a favorite book or Bible, or a pretty painting- any items that you find soothing or comforting.

Even with all these items, there will be days when unfinished business or errands will not allow you to settle your mind. When this happens, write the nagging thought on a pad of paper. Then, draw a line through the item. This will strike the item from your mind, while providing you with handy, still-legible reminder when your meditation time is through.

Meditation is the act of thinking of nothing. This isn't as easy as it sounds. During meditation we are quiet listeners and receptors for all the positive vibrations and information in the entire universe. When done consistently and properly, it can be vastly interesting and valuable.

Patients at the Whitewater and Sarasota centers gather at 7 p.m. each day to sit on a "magic carpet" and meditate together for a few minutes. This creates an atmosphere of mutual healing that helps each patient empty his mind and forget his problems. This is the "inner peace" that is so important for good health and vision.

Inhaling Health

Deep breathing is a kind of cleaning. It brings in new energy and fresh oxygen, while letting go stress, body tension and carbon dioxide waste. We teach a rhythmic abdominal breathing technique, and patients practice it from two to five minutes several times each day. It is also very useful for dealing with high stress situations.

One of the most important therapies I advise in the treatment and rehabilitation of patients' vision and health problems is the technique of "deep breathing" and "postures."

293

It is not a difficult act to master. Try these steps:

ABDOMINAL BREATHING

* Find a comfortable chair outdoors or in a well-ventilated room. Sit erect, with feet flat on the floor, hands resting in your lap. Wear loose, comfortable clothing.

* Inhale deeply through your nose, your mouth closed. Fill the bottom half of your lungs first, expanding your abdomen so your belly fills out like a balloon. Then, with no pause, let your breath fill the top half of your lungs, expanding your ribcage. Imagine the air swirling upward and around your heart cavity. Don't hold your breath or strain, or raise your shoulders.

* Then, smoothly and slowly exhale, using your abdominal muscles to flatten your belly last of all. Do not slouch forward on exhaling. You will notice after a few breaths that your "exhale muscles" seems to contract toward a point in the center of your chest. Concentrate on this spot as your breath in and out.

* With each intake of breath, visualize an intake of energy and life. With each exhale, imagine an outflow of toxins from the body. As you breathe, imagine oxygen being carried throughout your body, bathing your eyes, tissues and organs with life-giving nourishment. Feel your muscles loosen and tension ease.

294

If you find this exercise difficult, try reading one of the many good books on this special breathing technique available in certain "health improvement" stores. Practicing this breathing as well as special therapeutic postures should become a part of your daily life, even if it's only for a few moments each day.

It is especially important for elderly people to use their full lung capacity. They often sit for long periods of time, slouched into comfortable easy chairs. Unfortunately, these postures promote weak muscles of lungs and abdominal cavities. It's no wonder the elderly suffer from so many pulmonary illnesses, as their lower lungs stagnate with stale, uncirculated air. In extreme cases, fluid can build up there, providing a breeding ground for infection and bogging down basic life functions. These long sedentary conditions also interfere with the circulation of blood and oxygen reaching the eyes and brain due to gravity. Sit up straight during your television shows, and don't forget the many benefits of a daily stroll or a mild exercise session.

Once you've tried this breathing exercise, you have a potent weapon against the stress that may sometimes overwhelm you, especially if you tend to be hot tempered. When that annoying phone call comes, or someone puts one too many items into your "in basket, simply push your chair back and breathe. You'll be amazed at how this simple exercise can channel your negative energy into a positive, calm control of almost any situation.

SPECIFIC TREATMENTS

Macular Degeneration

Macular degeneration isn't an accurate term. This isn't really a disease or degeneration - it's a lowering of the functions of the macular cells, the cones inside the eye's retina. These cones suffer from poor blood circulation and oxygen deprivation.

It is popularly believed that cones (nerve cells in the eyes) cannot be improved once they are functioning at a lower level. But we have seen much success in using human-bio-feedback (visualization) to call on the body's "fibroblasts," universal cells that provide injured or diseased tissues with a rich new supply of capillaries, (tiny blood vessels), oxygen and nutrition.

You can give macular cells additional oxygen by doing deep breathing, and by bringing that oxygen through the blood vessels from the heart, the carotid arteries in the neck and its branches and the ophthalmic arteries to the eye. This carries more of the immune cells, leukocytes and oxygen to these tiny nerve cells (cones) that need it so much.

"The reason for (macular degeneration) is a lack of oxygen, lack of high class nutrition and nerve supply. All of these can be properly supplied by teaching the patient how to use his diaphragm, how to increase oxygen levels, and how to increase the amount of blood supply to his eyes by relaxing the blood vessel walls that lead to his neck and head."

Helen Bennett of Pennsylvania found much relief from her poor functioning cones through meditative practices. But when she became upset after a series of family crises, she began to see the results of her stress producing serious changes in her eyesight again.

"My vision was being affected, after I had such wonderful results," she wrote.

"However, control was regained after using the treatments that I learned at Dr. Salov's vision center in Whitewater, Wisconsin, and I continue to have improvement in my eyesight."

Not only do I teach patients to improve the amount of oxygen and blood circulation to their eyes, but I also teach them how to relax and improve their nutrition with natural, organic foods as well as how to relieve their daily stresses. Special tapes help them learn certain methods of relaxation and meditation.

CATARACT RELIEF

Cataracts are described in a foregoing chapter of this book, but a quick review will help clarify Dr. Salov's approach to this condition of the eyes which gradually reduces vision and leads to blindness.

The crystalline lens is pliable, soft surface that sits in the back of the eye, behind the iris.

It is encapsulated and bathed in a special fluid called "aqueous fluid," a clear substance that protects and gives nutrition to the crystalline lens. The lens, when it is healthy, can contract or expand to see objects that are far away or nearby. But as it ages, this lens tends to harden - with the resulting farsightedness that sets in at about age 40.

When the lens starts to become harder and dehydrates, it loses it's transparency. This condition is called "cataract." This often happens among diabetics, whose bodies cannot properly process sugars. With diabetics' poor general blood circulation, and the poor nutrition and sugar metabolism common in "developed societies," they are a prime candidate for cataracts.

Other causes of cataracts include the accumulation of cholesterol and poisonous, toxic materials such as camphor, asbestos fumes and environmental pollution. These produce cataracts which are not the same type, but are of special variety different from those produced by poor circulation, stresses and lack of good, clean oxygen.

A small percentage of cataract surgeries produce serious complications of infection, hemorrhage and retinal detachment, which sometimes causes complete blindness.

We have learned how to utilize our important immune cells. Our leukocytes are able to dissolve and completely absorb cataracts by methods of visualization (human-bio-feed-back) and additional therapies we teach at our vision centers. We have learned how to completely absorb cataracts by teaching our patients how to use visualization to guide special immune cells (leukocytes and fibroblasts) to absorb and completely remove the cataract material. Good vision results, and the cataract is taken care of without medicines or surgery.

DIABETIC RETINOPATHY
(See diagram on page 313)

Many diabetics suffer from diabetic retinopathy, a serious deterioration of vision of both young and old. Dr. Salov has done extensive research into this condition. It develops slowly, as thousands of tiny capillaries inside the eyeball break, hemorrhage and scar. Sometimes, they invade the vitreous humor (the transparent jello-like substance which fills about two-thirds of the inside of the eye), blocking the visual stimuli as it passes through the retina, causing poor vision, and eventually blindness.

Through years of research in European and American hospitals and universities, I concluded that diabetes is as much a disease of circulation as it is of metabolism.

Diabetes is a disease primarily of blood circulation throughout the entire body. Years before any sugar metabolism problems show themselves, tiny capillaries (the smallest blood vessels in our bodies) show changes of structure and evidence that the condition of diabetes starts at least ten years before any metabolic sugar test is positive.

Diabetic retinopathy is usually treated with laser surgery or vitrectomy, the removal of the vitreous matter in the eye. Both procedures are expensive and risky. They are absolutely useless, and do not improve the condition. The restored tissues soon begin again to be invaded by hemorrhages - evidence that the symptom was treated, not the cause.

I believe diabetic retinopathy can be prevented or alleviated, but the whole human organism must be considered. For the eyes to be healthy, the whole body must be healthy. Vision, one of Mankind's most priceless possessions, depends on a healthy body. Eyesight is a barometer of health.

Our treatments of this disease include a measured, carefully overseen withdrawal from all drugs, radical changes in eating habits, including fasting, juice therapies, and exclusion of all sugar, alcohol, coffee, tea, soda pop, tobacco, salt and white flour products. Therapeutic skin baths are applied, as well as light and cold therapies.

This intensive program concentrates on normalizing the diabetic's metabolism, establishing biochemical stability after years of artificial chemical influence, strengthening vital organs and re-establishing circulation.

IN SUMMARY

Cures are always accomplished by the body's own curative forces. Modern, natural, alternative eye care aims to discover the initial causes of ill health and loss of vision. Then, the physician must teach. "Teacher" is what "physician" really means- convince, inspire and instruct the patient about the changes that must take place in his environment, lifestyle and living habits to help him build his total health and vision.

We warn our patients not to pick and choose which parts of his therapy are most convenient or simple to apply - they must all work together to restore eye health.

In order to rehabilitate and rejuvenate people with poor vision and poor health, it is important and necessary to follow our entire program. It must also be appreciated that the development of "inner peace" is an important part of all therapies advised at our vision and health centers in Whitewater, Wisconsin and Sarasota, Florida. I recall a case with a young Italian man whose glaucoma symptoms were eradicated when he settled a long-standing feud with his family. "Inner peace" is essential before healing can begin. Inner peace is not a religious thing. It's a therapeutic thing.

Dr. Salov's success stories don't stop here. His therapies go beyond eyes, to cerebral palsy, brain hemorrhages, stomach ulcers and asthma. These short chapters can give you only a glance at the depth of his research and wisdom.

Those interested in details on Dr. Salov's therapies and clinical programs can contact him at:

> The Vision Health Center
> W3064 Piper Road
> Whitewater, Wisconsin 53190

Chapter 13

Envision
Great Vision

It is a documented fact that a large portion — up to 90 percent — of the brain remains unused over a lifetime. This vast, untapped power can be harnessed, and put to work to accomplish many wonders. Stroke victims, with therapy, can often train their brains to use new pathways for speech and motor functions when the old paths have been destroyed. If brain surgery severs important sensory nerves, other portions of the brain sometimes take over, and the patient miraculously recovers abilities he'd assumed were lost forever. Considering this, it shouldn't be surprising to learn that mind power can heal the body of many diseases.

Dr. Salov is a proven teacher of these therapies, which were outlined in the previous two chapters. One of his greatest success stories involves the four-year-old child whose photos appear on pages 311 and 312. This was a case of five hemangiomas, or "blood tumors," growing behind the left eyeball.

303

Children are particularly good subjects for visualization therapy, as their minds are not cluttered with negatives. Little Sara, despite her painful condition, proved a model patient.

One October evening, Sara's parents noticed her left eye was red and glassy, but thought she'd simply bumped it during the day's romping. But the eye didn't improve. Three days later, her eye was swollen and forcing itself from its socket — pushed forward almost an inch by the tumors growing in the space behind it. As days passed, Sara's eyesight deteriorated rapidly. Her ophthalmologist prescribed medication, but small hemorrhages occurred in her eye, preventing further chemical treatment.

Finally, the distraught parents were told the sad facts: The rapidly growing tumors were constricting the optic nerve and several vital blood vessels. The tumors could be surgically removed, but their daughter may lose her eye in the process.

Sara underwent three separate surgical procedures in order to remove the tumors in the back of her eye. Each of these procedures was unsuccessful. The surgeons were unable to remove the five tumors, even after they removed a portion of her temporal bone (a portion of her left cheek bone, called temporalectomy).

After these unsuccessful operations Sara's parents were advised that they would have to wait until the eyeball was completely out of the socket. Then the entire mass, the five tumors and the eyeball could be surgically removed. In time, healing would make possible an artificial glass eye, for cosmetic purposes.

Broken-hearted but still hopeful, Sara's parents attended a lecture they had read about on Modern, Alternative Ophthalmology, conducted by eye specialist, Leslie H. Salov, M.D., Director of the Jeanne Patterson Vision & Health Center in Whitewater, Wisconsin. After the lecture, Dr. Salov was given a brief description of Sara's medical history and present status and was asked if he knew of anything which may help the child. Dr. Salov agreed to help Sara, and her parents immediately took Sara to Dr. Salov's Center, where the doctor sat the child on his knee and gently explained just what her problem was.

He showed her how tumors grow, and used pictures and models to show her what would happen if the growth continued. To ensure her understanding, Dr. Salov asked Sara to draw a picture of the inside of her eye.

The picture arrived with Sara the next day, in bright crayon colors. An eye stood in the foreground, with an angry-looking face. Standing behind it were five dark shapes - the tumors. Dr. Salov was pleased at her elemental understanding of her condition, and set about helping the girl use *visual imagery* to relieve her own pain (visualization).

Dr. Salov and Sara's mother gave the girl a beaker of red-colored water and a plastic syringe. Dr. Salov told Sara to look at her eye picture and imagine the tumors were inside the bulb of the syringe. As she squeezed the red water out of the syringe, she imagined the tumors spurting out. As the bulb grew smaller, she imagined the tumors shrinking, until they disappeared.

In addition, we taught Sara how to utilize her very important immune cells in her bone marrow called leukocytes (white corpuscles). These leukocytes are live, motile cells which can migrate to any part of the body where they are needed by the commands of the individual (visualization).

These leukocytes are also cannibalistic, which means that they recognize when material in the body is foreign and not usable to the body. They produce a very potent enzyme called *Dis-mu-tase* which can secrete onto the tumors which dissolves them and helps the leukocytes to actually "eat" the tumors and destroy the actual tumor growths completely. Because leukocytes are motile, tiny pieces of these tumors can enter Sara's bloodstream and be carried to the lungs eventually and to the ends of the digestive tract and urinary organs. The material it has cannibalized then can be eliminated from the body completely.

We taught Sara how to use this marvelous human mechanism of her immune system and because of her great child-like imagination and desire to get well, she cooperated so wonderfully that eventually all of the five tumors were completely absorbed and eliminated from the back of her eye.

With dedicated repetition over a month's time, Sara's protruding left eye began to re-settle into its socket. The tumors began to absorb into Sara's bloodstream, with continued visual imagery over 11 months, Sara's vision was almost normal, and her pretty little face had lost its deformed look.

"We first saw Sara in November," Dr. Salov said. "Before the end of December, the absorption of the tumors from behind the eye, as well as the restoration and positioning of the eye to its normal orbital depth demonstrated, more than my description of words, the phenomenal, awesome power of the mind... and the too-often latent, unappreciated, God-given ability to heal ourselves."

Like several other noted visualization therapists, Dr. Salov developed his method himself, when he found his own eyesight failing. After being forced into retirement by a severe degenerative condition, Dr. Salov heard of visualization therapy — an idea he first pooh-poohed as totally outside the realm of science.

With nothing to lose, Dr. Salov began practicing visualization therapy on himself, at home. As his vision slowly recovered, Dr. Salov became convinced - and is today one of the therapy's strongest advocates.

How To Practice Visualization Therapy Getting Started On Your Own...

If you are unable to find a doctor or counselor to prepare a treatment plan for you that includes visualization techniques, you can develop your own.

First, acknowledge your disease as an unwelcome invader which should be eliminated. Imagine the "good guys," the lymphocytes and macrophage cells of your immune system, attacking and defeating the "bad guys," the diseased tissues. Don't be afraid to use silly images, or borrow characters from familiar stories, movies or television shows. Make a drawing of your "heroes" and "villains," as drawing makes the imagery become concrete. Don't worry if your artistic ability is zero, this picture is only for your use. Take your epitome of good — your White Knight or King David — and picture him attacking and overwhelming your Godzilla or Goliath.

You may want to add props, like Sara's syringe of water, to further impress your subconscious mind. These hands-on images can help even the rustiest imagination leap into the healing process.

One man had success against a tumor by slowly carving a monster-sized potato, sliver by tiny sliver, while visualizing an internal tumor being steadily carved away by a golden knife. Because visualization isn't by any means instantaneous, the man gradually started in on a slightly smaller potato, and continued the process daily to reinforce his healing imagery. (And perhaps all those nutritious hash-brown potatoes aided his recovery as well!)

Other patients do a series of daily drawings, showing their disease slowly yielding to a small, persistent, cartoon shape a sort of yellow Pac-man figure. Others opt to relax in a quiet place and concentrate on running mental images through their minds, over and over. The conquering hero vanquishing the dreaded enemy. Simply directing the immune system to marshal its forces and heal the specific eye condition can be equally effective, without outside props or artwork. The key is strong purposeful, powerful images, repeated consistently.

Twice A Day

Most authorities recommend practicing visualization for at least two 20-minute periods every day. During this time, concentrate intensely on the mental image of the disease, and its gradual easing. Once your mental images are strong, your subconscious will deliver them at will. At odd times through the day, call up the images to reinforce your immune system. It's also a good idea to begin and end the day with a few moments of focused visualization.

How long will it take? Who knows? The success of visualization therapy depends on many factors, including your commitment and ability to focus your subconscious onto the healing task. This is not a universally recognized medical procedure, but a great many cures have been documented using this method. Visualization therapy does work. If you decide to use this dynamic technique to eliminate disease and restore visual health, let us know of your experiences.

Proceed with caution — It is true that the mind possesses powers that science cannot explain, but it would be unwise in the extreme to rely solely on visualization techniques to treat eye ailments. Never put off consulting with a qualified doctor, or arbitrarily decide to discontinue treatment if you are under a doctor's care.

Sara's Eyes: A Miracle In Pictures

These photographs, as painfully graphic as they are, illustrate the dramatic reversal of Sara's eye condition.

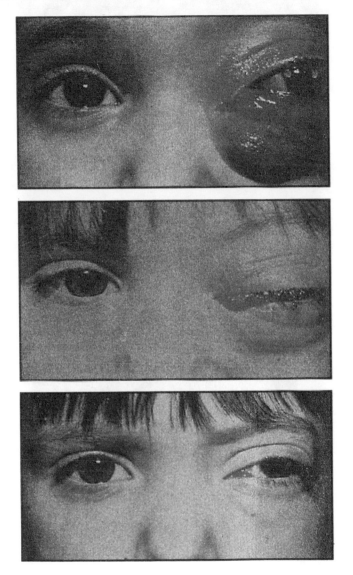

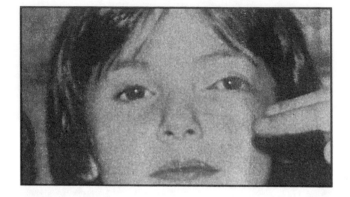

These illustrations aptly show the remarkable recovery experienced by this youngster and her fertile imagination.

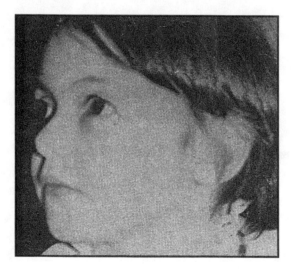

Diabetic Retinopathy
A Leading Cause of Blindness

These slides taken during a 20-year development of diabetes show the gradual development of *diabetic retinopathy*. (1) Normal blood circulation. The optic nerve head is in the center. (2) through (5) shows the progression of diabetic retinopathy and the final slide (6) shows extensive scarring and hemorrhaging. The person is blind.

Appendix I
Personal Statements

The following statements are from persons who have attended the intensive training and therapy Program.

All these people were told that nothing could be done to improve their vision or prevent further vision loss!

Macular Degeneration

"Upsetting occurrences have happened in my life since my last letter. My vision was being affected, after I had such wonderful results. However, control was regained by using your teachings learned in Whitewater, and I continue again to improve."

Helen Bennett, Pa.

Kerataconus

(Misshapen cornea resulting in extreme loss of vision) "As a 1st year Ophthalmological resident in a well known University Eye Training Center, I did not get results... They simply could not improve my vision. With trepidation I attended your Two-Week Program. I shall be everlastingly grateful to you and the Program for the good results I received."

J. Okunberg, M.D., La.

314

Glaucoma

"A dramatic improvement in my vision from 20/100 to 20/25. Thanks."

Gloria Swanson, N.Y. (1981)
and Hollywood, Ca.

Diabetic Retinopathy

"I couldn't believe it... getting improvement... the hemorrhages stopped and I can see better."

Goldstein, R., N.Y.

Burned Cornea

(Acid splashed in eyes) "I'd like to take this opportunity of our Thanksgiving to thank you for one of my greatest gifts. The restoration of my full vision can be attributed to only you and our Lord. I think of you often and wish you many more years of service to all who need your professional care. God Bless."

Ron Verhulst, D.D.S.

Cataract

"No one believed this... a man of 80, but thanks to you, Dr. Salov, my eyesight when I saw you was 20/100 in my right eye and 20/80 in my left eye. After spending 2 weeks with you and practicing what I learned for six months faithfully, my RE is 20/40 and LE 20/30 and I got my drivers license."

Hamilton Merrill, Mass.

315

Macular Degeneration

"I would like to report that my eyes continue to improve. I did regress a bit because we vacationed in Florida and were so busy I didn't continue your program. However, I did go to see Dr. Burke while you were in Europe. He feels my improvement is, in his words, "fantastic.""

"Buddy" Wheeler, Wis.

Glaucoma

"I must tell you the good news, my eye pressure is now 13-14, the lowest in many years. It usually runs 37-36. The two weeks with you made this difference."

M. Clark, Fla.

Retinitis Pigmentosa

"I feel I am making progress with the right eye and perhaps have stopped the deterioration in the left. While the trip to Whitewater was a hard one, it was worth it. Keep up the good work."

Paula Jackson, Ill.

Iritis

"Having suffered with this terrible condition, I came to you with little hope... but I cannot thank you and your Program enough for helping me to get back pretty much to normal eye health."

Penny Bruce, Wis.

Appendix II
Professional Presentations

Dr. Salov's research and work on "Visual Pathways Affecting the Whole Person" has been presented to:

University of Athens - Athens, Greece
3rd International Conference on Medicine of the
    Future - Arta, Greece
University of Berne - Switzerland
Hadassah Medical University - Israel
University of Alexandria - Egypt
Cunard Steamship Line (On Board the QE-2)
Walter Reed Army Medical Center
Michael Reese Hospital
University of Wisconsin
Duquesne University
University of Illinois
Beaver County Medical Society
Dane County Dept. of Social Services
Association Humanistic Psychology
International Cancer Association
Sarasota County Health Dept. - Nurse's Training
Florida Health Institute
National Health Federation
The Olive Garvey Center For Human Functioning
Manatec College
National Health Expo
South Central Florida Health Systems Council
Consumers Health Organization of Canada
American Hygiene Society
Palmer College of Chiropractic
5th International Congress Himalayan Institute
Wisconsin Student Association
Whole Health Institute
Hippocrates World Health

317

Appendix III
Biography of Leslie H. Salov, M.D.

Education

Bachelor of Science (B.S.) - Upsala College, East Orange, N.J.

Doctor of Optometry (O.D.) - Pennsylvania College of Optometry, Philadelphia, Pa.

Doctor of Medicine & Surgery (M.D.) - University of Berne, Faculty of Medicine, Berne Switzerland

Doctor of Philosophy (Ph.D.) - University of Zurich, Zurich Switzerland

Internship

Morristown Memorial Hospital, Morristown, N.J.

Residency In Specialty of Ophthalmology

Montefiore Hospital, Department of Ophthalmology, Pittsburgh, Pa.

Eye and Ear Hospital, University of Pittsburgh, Pittsburgh, Pa.

Additional Background

Staff Physician: New Jersey State Mental Hospital, Greystone Park, N.J.

Primary Researcher: Research Program- "Diabetic Retinopathy, Its Diagnosis & Treatment" Montefiore Hospital, Pittsburgh, Pa.

Awarded a travel-research grant from the Bernard Baruch Medical Foundation to study at the following clinics in Europe:
University of Leiden, Holland
University of Rotterdam, Holland
University of Ghent, Belgium

318

University of Zurich, Switzerland
St. Gallen Institute, St. Gallen, Switzerland
University of Athens, Greece
University of Berne, Switzerland

Primary Researcher and Consultant for the Atomic Energy Commission in a study involving over 5000 men to determine the reaction to the eyes from exposure to radiation while working in the construction of nuclear sites throughout the United States

Instructor - Post Graduate Congress: Slit-lamp Microscopy & Eye Surgery, Montefiore Hospital, Pittsburgh, Pa.

Post Graduate Studies, Armed Forces Institute of Pathology, Washington, D.C.

Guest Lecturer, Department of Philosophy: Instituto Allende, University of Guanajuata, San Miguel de Allende, Mexico

Independent study and research to clinics:
University of Budapest, Hungary
University of Yugoslavia, Dubrovnick, Yugoslavia
Oxford University, Oxford, England

Associate Professor of Philosophy and Psychology, Rutgers University, New Jersey

Guest Lecturer with Carlton Fredericks, Ph.D., International Nutrition Authority, on his broadcasts as far back as 1947

Director, New Jersey Health Association

Invited by Dr. Paavo Airola, international nutritionist, to write foreword to his book *Are You Confused?*

Active practice of medicine and surgery through 1975

Faculty member of Himalayan International Institute; Swami Rama, Founder and Spiritual Leader; Branches in major cities of the United States and abroad

Frequent guest speaker on major radio and TV stations

Lectures to and conducts and coordinates Programs in Wholistic Health for major Universities, State Agencies, Executive Personnel in Industry, Service Clubs, etc., using Alternative Methodologies: Nutrition, Yoga, Meditation, Biofeedback, Visualization, Chromography, etc., synthesized with Western Medical Science

Member: American Holistic Medical Association, International Academy of Biological Medicine, Academy of Preventive Medicine

Director, **The Vision and Health Center**, Whitewater, Wisconsin, a center dedicated to Improving Health and Vision, using the eyes as the "opening" to the "body and whole person."

Publications

"Treatment of the Partially Blind"

"Visual Therapy for the Cerebral Palsied Child"

"Diabetes and Retinal Changes"

"Herzglykoside und Kohlenhydratstoffwechsel" (in German)

"Medical Missiles"

Numerous papers to medical journals

Forworded William L. Fischer's book *"How To Fight Cancer And Win,"* 1994 Edition, also listed on back cover endorsement as well as contributed important information relative to the therapeutic usage of "visualization" or "Human-bio-feed-back" which is used for serious eye problems and diseases.

320

Appendix IV

Other Conditions Affecting the Eye

There are many disorders and diseases which may affect any area of the eye, from the lid to the optic nerve. Some of these, naturally, are more common than others. If you believe that you may have any of these conditions which we outline here, consult your opthalmologist immediately.

Blepharitis. This condition may be associated with allergies and dandruff scales. It is characterized by an inflammation of the lid margin, redness and swelling. In its mild form, there is a crusting of the lash bases. Some lashes may fall out, but others grow back to replace them. However, in the more severe form, the lashes do not grow back and the lid margin is distorted.

Internal Hordeolum or Stye. An infection of a gland on the *underside* of the lid.

External Hordeolum or Stye. An infection of a hair follicle, similar to a boil. It begins with a general swelling and pain on the lid. It then localizes into a red area with a yellowish center at the lid margin. Eventually, it breaks open to dishcarge pus and heals quickly.

Chalazion. A chronic and sometimes inflammatory enlargement of the lid gland. Usually a painless condition, it appears as a bump or swelling and gradually increases in size.

Entropian. The lid margin turns inward which causes the lashes to rub, irritating the cornea. This occurs most often in older people or after an injury or a burn.

Ptosis. A drooping of the upper lid, seen mostly in older

people who suffer from a loss of muscle tone. It may also be due to a congential condition caused by a paralysis of the lid muscles and a neurological disorder.

Ectropion. A condition where the lid margin turns outward, producing excessive tearing as well as itching and burning of the exposed inner lid. This, too, usually occurs in the elderly because of the loss of the muscle tone.

The Conjunctiva

Hemorrhage. A spontaneous hemorrhage may occur on the white of the eye giving it a bright, blood red appearance. It may be caused by coughing, sneezing or by rubbing the eyes too hard.

Pterygium. This condition is a triangular shaped, elevated, vascular tissue on the white of the eye. It is only a danger if it grows across the cornea and blocks sight.

Pinguecula. A harmless, small, yellowish elevation of the white of the eye, normally found on the nasal side. It becomes more noticeable with age.

Optic Nerve

Retroblubar Neuritis. An inflammation of the optic nerve, usually accompanied by painful eye movements and loss of central vision.

Optic Atrophy. Destruction of the optic nerve fibers due to disease, injury, or pressure directly on the nerve. Portions of central or side vision are lost with this condition.

322

The Retina

Choroiditis. An inflammation of the choroid, affecting the overlying retina. Caused by a systemic disease which is often difficult to identify. The inflammatory lesions may be on one side and cause little trouble with vision. However, if it is near the macula, loss of sight will occur. While the inflammation slowly subsides, repeated attacks are not uncommon.

Papillitis. An inflammation of the optic nerve disc.

Retinal Degeneration. Dengenerating changes usually caused by a disturbance in the vascular system. This condition usually affects older people and will gradually reduce vision.

Arterial/Venous Occlusion. There are two areas where this can occur:

Central Retinal Artery. Obstruction here or in a principal branch will cause a loss of vision. If the main artery is affected, vision loss is total, otherwise only the area supplied by the branch will be affected.

Major Vein. Causes muscle hemorrhaging and sight impairment. As the hemorrhage is slowly absorbed, vision will gradually improve.

Arteriosclerosis. The arterial walls thicken, which restricts the flow of blood. As the condition becomes worse, small hemorrhages sometimes occur. It's possible, as a consequence of this condition, for an obstruction of a main artery or vein to occur.

Hypertensive Retinopathy. This is caused by high blood pressure, which affects the retinal vessels. Besides arteriosclerosis, edema and hemorrhages may occur. The extent of vision loss is determined by the site and amount of retinal damage.

Sclera

Episcleritis. An inflammation of the loose connective tissue of the sclera. In appearance, it closely resembles conjunctivitis, except this condition is mostly restricted to a small area and is a deep red or purple in color.

Staphyloma. A small pigmented bulge in the white of the eye which is caused by a thinning of the sclera.

Vitreous

Muscae Volimtantes or Floaters. These are small, solidified particles which float in the vitreous and are seen as spots, threads or specks when one looks at a bright background. This is a harmless condition.

Lens

Subluxated Lens. In this condition, the lens is shifted out of its normal position, usually downward. The problem may be congenital or it could be the result of an injury. The degree of displacement determines whether vision is affected.

Iris

Iritis. An inflammation of the iris and of its ciliary body to which the iris is anchored. This condition causes pain and redness. The pupil is contricted and irregulraly shaped and the person will be extremely snesitive to light.

Iridodonesis. In this disorder, the iris trembles or quivers due to either a displaced or missing lens.

Heterochromia. A condition in which the iris of one eye differs in color from that of the other eye. Usually considered congenital, this condition is harmless. A recent color change is associated with iritis.

Coloboma. A congenital defect in which part of the iris is missing. It may also develop after eye surgery or an injury to the eye.

Synechiae. The condition is characterized by the iris adhering to the lens. Usually this develops after one has iritis. It is a painful problem and will produce an odd-shaped pupil. In some instances, the iris may also adhere to the back of the cornea following an eye injury or surgery.

Cornea

Abrasion. A breakdown of the surface layer of the cornea, which is accompanied by pain, tearing and light sensitivity. It is most often caused by injury of excessive contact lens wear.

Arcus Senilis. This condition, which is very common in older folks, produces a gray or whitish partial or full ring around the edge of the cornea. It is not a dangerous development.

Keratitis. An inflammation of the cornea, which may be either superficial or deep. With the superficial kind, the infection begins on the surface and is caused by an outside source. Various ulcerations may occur, depending upon the infecting agent, which will leave opaque scars after the eye heals.

The deep type of keratitis is tranmitted via the bloodstream and is most often confined to the inner layers. Most commonly, it is caused by congenital syphyllis and will appear in children and teenagers.

Ulceration. An erosion of the corneal surface, this problem is caused by bacteria, fungus, or a virus. It always causes scarring and in extreme cases may perforate through the entire cornea.

Vascularization. This condition occurs when the blood vessels invade the cornea—an area usually devoid of any vessels. It is caused by disease, injury or an inflammation.

Orbit

Enophthalmos. This looks as if the person has a sunken eyeball and usually occurs following an injury or in older people when portion of the fatty tissue is absorbed.

Exophthalmos. The problem of bulging eyes, it is caused by an over-active thyroid gland when both eyes are affected. When only one eye is involved, it may be caused by a tumor, an inflammation or a vascular condition.

Miscellaneous

Dacryocystitis. An infection of the tear drainage sac, which is located near the inner corner of the eye. A mild infection involves redness and slight swelling; more severe cases will cause pain and more obvious swelling.

Appendix V

Glossary of Selected Definitions

Accommodation: The process in which the shape of the lens of the eye adjusts for near vision so that light rays from a near external object are brought to a point of focus on the retina by the accommodated lens or the ciliary muscles around the eye.

Allergic Conjunctivitis: An inflammation of the conjunctiva in response to an allergy-causing substance.

Amblyopia: A failure of normal visual development in an eye without pathological defect and with the anatomical potential for normal vision.

Ametropia: Optical error; a condition in which faulty refraction of light rays prevents an image from being brought to focus on the retina, as in the case of myopia, hyperopia, or astigmatism.

Anisometropia: A condition in which the optics of one eye differ greatly from those of the other eye.

Anterior Chamber: The space behind the cornea and in front of the iris that is filled with aqueous fluid.

Aphakia: Absence of the crystalline lens in a human eye due to congenital, traumatic, pathological or some other cause.

Aqueous Fluid: Also called aqueous humor; the watery fluid that fills the anterior and posterior chambers of the eye; acts to nourish and lubricate the lens and cornea as well as to maintain the eyeball's consistency.

Astigmatism: An optical error characterized by an unequal curvature in one or more of the eye's refractive surfaces, most commonly the cornea, causing an object to come to focus at two points on the visual axis instead of coming to focus at one point.

Binocular Vision: Vision achieved when both eyes function together; one of the components of normal vision.

Biomicroscope: Also called a slit lamp; an optical instrument that isolates enlarged and illuminated sections of certain anatomical structures in the eye by utilizing a thin beam of light; particularly useful in examination of the anterior anatomy of the eye as well as the optical media.

Canal of Schlemm: Irregular space in the sclerocorneal region of the eye.

Cataract: A loss of transparency of any degree and for any reason in the lens of the eye.

Cones: Specialized cells of the retina sensitive to color and light intensity; important in light adaptation and color perception.

Contact Lens: A pair of small optical lenses generally made of plastic that correct optical defects inconspicuously by resting directly on the tear layer of the cornea.

Convex Lens: A lens of which one or both surfaces are curved outward. A concave lens curves inward.

Cornea: The curved, transparent membrane forming the front one-sixth of the outer coat of the eyeball; serves primarily as protection and is the outermost refractive surface of the eye.

Corneal Contact Lenses: Contact lenses that are fitted exclusively on the corneal surface; the most commonly used contact lenses today are corneal contact lenses.

Corneal Transplant: A surgical procedure in which a portion of clear donor cornea is used to replace a corresponding portion of the patient's opacified cornea.

Diopter: The unit used to measure the light-bending power of a lens.

Diplopia: Double vision; a pathological condition of vision in which a single object is perceived as two.

Distance Vision: Use of the eyes to view objects in the distance. Theoretically, that distance is infinity; the ophthalmological measurement of distance vision is made twenty feet from the eye; in practical terms, one uses distance vision to view anything that is beyond what is considered middle distance.

Emmetropia: The normal optical condition of the eye that permits rays of light to focus accurately on the retina.

Epikeratophakia: An operative procedure that changes the shape of the front surface of the eye and allows it to see well without the need of contact lenses and, in many cases, spectacles.

Eye Bank: A medical facility that keeps eyes removed from deceased donors to be used in corneal transplantation.

Farsighted Astigmatism: A type of astigmatism in which both points of focus have not yet been reached when light rays arrive at the retina.

Fibroblasts: Any cell or corpuscle from which connective tissue is developed.

Focus: The point at which light rays meet after passing through a refractive surface.

Fovea Centralis: The small, normal anatomical depression located in the center of the macula.

329

Glaucoma: Disease of the eye characterized by increase in intraocular pressure (within your eyeball) which results in deterioration of the optic nerve and blindness.

Homeopathy: A system of medical treatments offering gentle stimulation of the body's inner healing resources. It uses remedies, which in larger doses, would produce symptoms of the disease. Used in minute portions, at times so small no molecule of the original substance remains, it relieves the symptoms.

Hypermetropia: A condition of farsightedness in a person designated a hypermetrope, which has him or her look into the distance without seeing clearly when the eye is at rest, because the image has not yet focused on the retina; also known as hyperopia.

Hyperopia: Commonly called farsightedness; the same optical error as hypermetropia in which an image has not yet come to a point of focus when it reaches the retina.

Interstitial Keratitis: An inflammation of the deeper layers of the cornea, causing clouding of the cornea.

Intraocular Pressure: The degree of firmness of the eyeball as controlled by secretion and drainage of aqueous fluid.

Iris: A disc-like diaphragm that is continuous in back with the ciliary body and is perforated in the center by the pupil; composed of vascular and muscular tissue, the latter controlling the size of the pupil. The color of the iris determines the color of an individual's eyes.

Iritis: Any inflammation of the iris.

Irregular Astigmatism: An unusual type in which the unequal curvature of the cornea causes an image to be focused at more than two points along the visual axis.

Keratoconus: A cone-shaped protrusion of the center of the cornea caused by a progressive thinning of the corneal tissue layers because of a structural weakness; its effects are highly irregular astigmatism and eventual rupture of the cornea if untreated.

Keratometer: An optical instrument used to measure the curvature of the cornea; of particular use in the fitting of contact lenses.

Keratomileusis: A refractive surgical procedure which splits a patient's cornea with a calibrated instrument called a microkeratome, removing that cornea's top layer, and reshaping it on a cryolathe, to reattach it without the addition of any donor material. This technique is the newest technology for correcting high myopia and/or aphakia.

Keratophakia: An operation for conditions of refraction involving the splitting of a patient's cornea in half with a calibrated instrument and lathing a donor cornea for placement between the two halves of the patient's operated cornea.

Laser: A powerful, concentrated beam of light that can generate a tiny, specified area; can be used in eye surgery. Some lasers cause tissues simply to atomize with very little heat produced.

Lens (Optical): A Transparent substance, usually made of glass or plastic, with two opposed surfaces, used to bend light and thereby change the point at which light rays focus, such as is used in the correction of optical errors.

Lens (Crystalline): A transparent, flexible body, convex on both surfaces and lying directly behind the iris of the eye; serves to focus the rays of light on the retina.

Leukocyte: White blood corpuscles. They have the power to ingest particulate substances. They are important in both defensive and reparative functions of the body.

Myopia: Commonly called nearsightedness; the optical error in which an object comes to a point of focus before it reaches the retina and is, thus, out of focus on the retina.

Nearsighted Astigmatism: Astigmatism in which both points of focus are in front of the retina.

Normal Vision: Two eyes with 20/20 visual acuity and fully developed binocularity.

Nystagmus: An involuntary, rhythmical oscillation of the eyeballs in a horizontal, vertical, or rotary direction; may be caused by a central (neurological) problem or a localized eye problem, and can either cause or result from faulty visual development.

Ophthalmologist: An eye surgeon, also called an oculist; a medical doctor trained in the diagnosis and treatment of eye diseases and correction of optical errors.

Ophthalmoscope: An instrument equipped with a system of mirrors and lights used to examine inside the eye.

Optic Nerve: The nerve of sight; the collection of specialized nerve fibers derived from the retina which unite and send visual impulses to the brain.

Optician: A specialist who makes eyeglasses in accordance with a doctor's prescription.

Optometrist: A doctor of optometry (O.D.) who is trained to test the eyes for nonmedical defects of vision in order to prescribe and dispense corrective lenses and to assist the patient in performing functional eye exercises.

Oxygen-Permeable Contact Lenses: Also called gas-permeable contact lenses; a type of contact that permits the exchange of oxygen through the lens material itself.

Pink Eye: Also known as conjunctivitis, any inflammation of the conjunctiva, which is the mucous membrane covering the exposed front portion of the sclera and continuing to form the lining of the inside of the eyelids.

Presbyopia: The normal physiological change in the ability to focus on near objects which occurs throughout life, normally becomes symptomatic in the forties and results in total loss of ability to focus on near objects around age 60; it does require correction with reading glasses. The condition results from the increased inelasticity in the crystalline lens of the eye.

Progressive Myopia: The tendency of nearsightedness to worsen during the growth period or over time as a result of some underlying pathological problem.

Refraction: The eye examination which determines the degree and nature of an optical error present plus the correction of the error.

Retinia: The thin, delicate, transparent sheet of nervous tissue that lines the back two-thirds of the eyeball; functions as the receptor of visual stimuli, which it transmits to the brain via the optic nerve.

Retinitis Pigmentosa: A rare disease characterized by chronic and progressive degeneration of the retinal pigmentation; hereditary in nature, usually results in little or no vision by middle age; night blindness is an early symptom.

Rods: Specialized cells of the retina sensitive to low intensities of light and important in dark adaptation.

Sclera: The curved, opaque, protective white layer forming the back five-sixths of the outer coat of the eyeball; the white of the eye.

Tonometer: An instrument used to measure intraocular pressure; a principal part of diagnostic screening for glaucoma.

20/20 Vision: The expression of visual acuity indicating that the test subject can see at 20 feet what a normal seeing person sees at 20 feet; one of the components of normal vision; also expressed as 6/6 to represent six meters rather than 20 feet.

Visual Acuity: The sharpness of vision as determined by a comparison with normal optical ability to define certain letters at a given distance, usually 20 feet.

Appendix VI

Sources of Herbs and Herb Products

CALIFORNIA
Herbs of Mexico
3859 Whittier Blvd.
Los Angeles, CA 90023
Tel. (213) 221-0064

Kitazawa Seed Co.
356 W. Taylor St.
San Jose, CA 95110
Tel. (408) 292-4420
(Seeds)

Lhasa Karnak Herb Co.
2513 Telegraph Ave.
Berkeley, CA 94704
Tel. (415) 548-0380
(Herbs, teas, spices)

Nature's Herb Company
281 Ellis St.
San Francisco, CA 94102
Tel. (415) 474-2756
(Herbs, herbal preparations)

Organic Foods & Gardens
4177 W. 3rd St.
Los Angeles, CA 90040
Tel. (213) 386-1440
(Herbs, etc.)

CONNECTICUT
Capriland's Herb Farm
Silver St.
Coventry, CT 06238
Tel. (213) 742-7244
(Herbs)

IDAHO
Lewiston Health Food
Center
861 Main
Lewiston, ID 83501
Tel. (208) 799-3100
(Herbs)

ILLINOIS
Dr. Michael's Herb Products
5109 North Western Ave.
Chicago, IL 60625
Tel. (312) 271-7738
(Herb products)

Kramer's Health Food
Store
29 East Adams St.
Chicago, IL 60603
Tel. (312) 922-0077
(Herbs)

INDIANA
Indiana Botanic Gardens, Inc.
Box 5
Hammond, IN 46325
Tel. (219) 947-4040
(Herbs, herb preparations, gums, oils, resins)

Moses J. Troyer
Lone Organic Farm
Route 1, Box 58
Millersburg, IN 46543
Tel. (219) 642-3385
(Herbs)

KENTUCKY
Ferry-Morse Seed Co.
Box 200
Fulton, KY 42041
Tel. (502) 472-3400
(Herbs, seeds)

MAINE
Conley's Garden Center
Boothbay Harbor, ME 04538
Tel. (207) 633-5020
(Wildflowers, ferns, garden plants)

MARYLAND
Carroll Gardens
P.O. Box 310
East Main St.
Westminster, Md 21157
Tel. 1-800-638-6334
(Herbs)

NEW JERSEY
Le Jardin du Gourmet
Box 245
Ramsey, NJ 07446
Tel. (201) 891-2070
(Herbs, spices, seeds)

NEW YORK
Kalustyan Orient Export Trading Corp.
123 Lexington Ave.
New York, NY 10016
Tel. (212) 685-3416

Kiehl Pharmacy
109 Third Ave.
New York, NY 10003
Tel. (212) 475-3400
(Herbs, spices)

NORTH CAROLINA
Wilcox Drug Co., Inc.
P.O. Box 391
Boone, NC 28607
Tel. (704) 264-3615
(Herbs)

OREGON
Nichols Garden Nursery
1190 North Pacific High-
way
Albany, OR 97321
Tel. (503) 928-9280
(Herbs, spices, seeds,
plants)

PENNSYLVANIA
Haussman's Pharmacy
6th & Girard Ave.
Philadelphia, PA 19127
Tel. (215) 627-2143
(Herbs, mixtures, oil,
gums)

Penn Herb Company
603 N. 2nd St.
Philadelphia, PA 19123
Tel. (215) 925-3336
(Herbs)

Tatra Herb Company
222 Grove St.
Morrisville, PA 19067
Tel. (215) 722-5305
(Herbs)

RHODE ISLAND
Green Herb Gardens
Greene, RI 02827
Tel. (401) 397-3652
(Fresh and dried herbs,
teas, seeds)

Meadowbrook Herb Garden
Route 138
Wyoming, RI 02898
Tel. (401) 539)-7603 or
    1-800-253-5005
(Herbs, herb products,
spices)

TENNESSEE
Savage Farm Nursery
Box 125
McMinnville, TN 37110
Tel. (615) 668-8902
(Wildflowers, garden
plants)

VERMONT
Putney Nursery, Inc.
Box 13
Putney, VT 05346
Tel. (802) 387-5577
(Wildflowers)

Vermont Country Store
Weston, VT 05161
Tel. (802) 824-3184
(Herbs, spices, condiments,
grains)

WASHINGTON
Cedarbrook Herb Farm
Route 1, Box 1047
Sequim, WA 98382
Tel. (206) 683-7733
(Herb plants)

WISCONSIN
Northwestern Processing
Co.
217 North Broadway
Milwaukee, WI 53202
Tel. (414) 276-1031
(Herbs, teas, nuts, spices)

Olds Seed Co.
Box 1069
Madison, WI 53701
Tel. (608) 221-9877

CANADA
World-Wide Herb Ltd.
11 S. Catherine St. East
Montreal 129, Quebec
Tel. (514) 842-1838
(Herbs)

Appendix VII

Homeopathic Organizations

The following is a list of homeopathic organizations which can supply you with information about homeopathy.

National Center for Homeopathy
1500 Massachusetts Avenue, NW
Washington, DC 20005

American Institute of Homeopathy
1500 Massachusetts Avenue, NW
Washington, DC 20005

United States Homeopathic Association
6560 Backlick Road
Springfield, VA 22150

International Foundation for Homeopathy
1141 NW Market Street
Seattle, WA 98107

Liga Medicorm Homeopathica Internationalis
(The International League of Homoeopathic Medicine)
P.O. Box 66
A.B. Blowmendaal, The Netherlands

Pan-American Homeopathic Medical Congress
Francisco del Paso y Troncoso Edificio 166
Entrada D. Unidad Kennedy
Mexico 9, D.F.

British Homeopathic Association
27A Devonshire Street
London, WIN 1RJ, England

Sources of Homeopathic Medicines

Homeopathic medicines are available in some health food stores. However, if you cannot find a store near you which carries these remedies there are several suppliers nationwide which you may contact. Below is a list of some of the major sources. All of the bussiness listed below offer active and realiable mail-order services.

They also carry homeopathic kits, which contain a variety of medicines for various problems.

Boericke and Tafel, Inc.
1011 Arch Street
Philadelphia, PA 19107

**John A. Bornemann
and Sons**
1208 Amosland Road
Norwood, PA 19074

Ehrhart and Karl, Inc.
17 N. Wabash Avenue
Chicago, IL 60602

HRI-Dolisos
6125 Tropicana Avenue
Las Vegas, NVf 89103

**Homeopathic Educational
Services**
2124 Kittredge Street
Berkeley, CA 94704

**Humphreys Pharmacal
Company***
63 Meadow Road
Rutherford, NJ 07070

**Luyties Pharmaceutical
Company**
4200 Laclede Avenue
St. Louis, MO 63108

**Standard Homeopathic
Pharmacy**
204-210 W. 131st Street
Los Angeles, CA 90061

**Washington Homeopathic
Pharmacy**
4914 Delray Avenue
Bethesda, MD 20814

*This pharmacy primarily sells combination medicines.

BIBLIOGRAPHY

Adams, Ruth and Frank Murray; *MegavitaminTherapy*, Larchmont Books, New York, 1974.

Benner, Dr. Maurice; *Vitamin A*, Alive Books, Vancouver, British Columbia, 1981.

Clark, Linda; *Secrets of Heath and Beauty*, The Devin-Adair Co., New York, 1969.

Clark, Linda, *Handbook of Natural Remedies for Common Ailments*, Devin-Adair Co. Old Greenwich Conn. 1976.

Consumer Reports, Editors of; *The Medicine Show*, Con sumer Union and the Untied States,

Inc., Mt. Vernon, New York, 1974. Deimal, Diana, *Vision Victory*, Chairu Publications, Pasadena Calif., 1980.

Duarte, Dr. Alex; *Cataract Breakthrough*, International Institute of Natural Health Sciences, Inc., Huntington Beach, Calif. 1982.

Fischer, William L.; *Miracle Healing Through Nature's Pharmacy*, Fischer Publishing Co., Canfield, Ohio 1986.

_____; *How to Fight Cancer and Win*, Fischer Publishing, Co., Canfield, Ohio 1987, 1994

_____; *Hidden Secretes of Super Perfect Health at Any Age*, Book, II, Fischer Publishing Co., Canfield, Ohio 1986

_____; *Throw Away Your Eyeglasses and Contact Lenses*, Fischer Publishing Co., Canfield, Ohio 1985.

Hoopes, Ann and Towsend, *Eye Power*, Alfred A. Knopf, New York, 1979.

Jones, William B., *The Natural Way to Good Vision Without Glasses*, Showcase books, Warren, Ohio 1977.

Hurdle, Dr. J. Frank, *A Country Doctor's Common Sense Health Manual*, Parker Publishing Co., Inc. West Nyack, New York, 1975.

Kavner, O.D., Richard S., and Lorraine Dusky, *Total Vision*, A & W Publishers, Inc. New York, 1978.

Mervyn, Leonard, *The Dictionary of Vitamins*, Thorsons
  Publishers, Inc., New York, 1984.
Rubman, M.D., Robert H. and Howard Rothman, *Future
  Vision*, Dodd Mead and Co., New York, 1987.
Thayer, Robert E., "Energy Walks," *Psychology Today*, Oct.
  1988. pp. 12-13.
Treben, Maria, *Health Through God's Pharmacy*, Wilhelm
  Ensthaler, Austria, 1984.
Walker, DPM, Morton, *The Doctor Rinse Formula*, Devin-
  Adair, Old Greenwich, Conn. 1983.
Zinn, O.D., Walter and Herbert Solomon, *The Complete
  Guide to Eye Care, Eyeglasses and Contact Lenses*,
  Frederick Fell Publishers, Inc. Hollywood, Fla., 1986.

INDEX

N

O

P